PARENTAL DEMENTIA

A GUIDE THROUGH ALL THE DIFFICULT QUESTIONS

The ESSENTIAL BOOK *for* DEMENTIA FAMILIES

BY KEITH GALAS WITH HALLE ESKEW

Parental Dementia: *A Guide through all the Difficult Questions*
© 2019 by Keith Galas with Halle Eskew

ISBN (Print): 978-1-54397-236-8
ISBN (eBook): 978-1-54397-237-5

Forward

Dementia.

Just hearing that word scares us to death. We begin thinking about loss, what we are going to lose and what the person with dementia is going to lose.

Next come the questions. What are we going to do? Where is my loved one going to live? Who is going to take care of them? Who is going to help me?

As you go through the disease process with someone, you begin to focus on what your loved one can't do. The negative side of life looms large.

Then, there are the behaviors. You simply cannot understand why someone would not want to take a shower and would actually hit you because you tried to give them one.

Even if you feel totally alone and think that you are the only one going through this, you are not alone. There are so many people and places that can help. Keith Galas is one of those people here to help.

This book is one of those great resources for help, and it contains so much useful information. His knowledge of what you are going through and his special ability to know what you need before you do is a true blessing.

I am a board certified geriatric pharmacist, specializing in Alzheimer's and other dementias, and have been a consultant pharmacist in long-term care communities for the better part of 28 years. I work with Keith and his team, and I can tell you that this book will be a comfort, help, and guide to you as you begin your journey with Parental Dementia. You can get your questions answered; you can learn to focus on the positive of what your loved one can do, and you can begin to understand some of the why's of behaviors.

Thank you, Keith, for your hard work and dedication to all of those affected by this horrible disease.

Lori Newcomb, RPh, BCGP

Introductions

Keith Galas

As a Memory Care Director, I've spent close to 20 years helping families work through the often heart-wrenching questions that rush upon them when they discover their loved one has dementia. What do I do now? Who will take care of Mom? How much will it cost for her care? How can I keep her safe?

My hope is that this book will ease the uncertainty and anguish I've seen in hundreds of families as they share their personal stories. Sadly, these accounts are increasing as dementia cases are on the rise. Roughly 10 percent of those over the age of 65 in the United States have Alzheimer's, and it is the sixth leading cause of death, according to the Alzheimer's Association.[1] There are more than 5 million Americans currently living with dementia. Unless a cure is found, as many as 16 million Americans could have dementia by 2050. Globally there are 50 million estimated dementia cases and, to that number, 10 million are added annually.[2] If you are about to embark on the road of caring for a loved one with dementia, you can be assured that you are not alone. Millions of family members have faced the same questions you may now be asking.

For many years, families have sat down with me to ask advice concerning their loved ones situation. I noticed that their questions and concerns are usually very similar. I wanted to write a book that answered those frequently asked dementia care questions. Each chapter of this book addresses a question that I hear most often.

Chapter 12 asks the question, "What should I expect from the community after we move in?" Which is a common question I receive after a family moves their loved one into my community. I thought who better to answer that chapter's question than one of our community's families. After some thought, I approached a family and asked if they would be willing to write a chapter in my book about their experiences. We set up a meeting and to my surprise I discovered someone that had an incredible insight for the dementia process, who was passionate about helping other families, and is also a very gifted writer. Therefore, I asked Halle Eskew to help me with this chapter. Halle agreed and also surprised me with writing a few stories of her family's journey with her mother and father's dementia.

I also decided to add a few of my own personal stories and include a few industry secrets that may save you time and money. For continuity, I decided to refer to Mom as the reader's loved one suffering from dementia, rather than your dad, sister, brother, husband or wife.

Ultimately, I wanted to write a book to help families understand that there is a way to get through this difficult time. No matter your life situation, I hope that this book will be used as a roadmap to help with the very difficult questions that you are about to encounter.

WHEN MY FAMILY NEEDED HELP

Before I became a care professional, I owned and operated a restaurant in Flagstaff, Arizona, about 150 miles from where my mother and father had retired. My father was diagnosed with Parkinson's and was experiencing the normal tremors and loss of balance associated with that condition. My mother was doing her best to be the at-home caregiver. One of the issues that many spouse caregivers are not trained for is that many people living with Parkinson's also experience sundowning and hallucinations.

One day my mother left my father at home to run to the store for groceries. She was gone no more than an hour. On her arrival back, she was greeted with police cars and a fire truck. Apparently, my father became very agitated and hallucinated that people were trying to break into the house. He then went outside and started yelling for these "people" to go away. The neighbors then called 911 and the ambulance, fire trucks, and police arrived. The police were very upset with my mother and they warned her that next time they would arrest her for leaving her at-risk husband alone.

So help was added to my father's daily care. I remember feeling guilty, skeptical, and untrusting. I never expected someone would be able to care for my father adequately. I was amazed watching a homecare caregiver treat my father with so much love and respect.

I am reminded of that day in a positive way as I watch my current care team. The passion and kindness that our care angels have for our residents and families is truly an inspiration. It takes me back to when I was one of the families just hoping for some help and receiving more than I could ever have anticipated.

–Keith

Halle Eskew

Our family journey into dementia care began with my dad, and later included my mom. They both went on to suffer the heartbreaking losses caused by Alzheimer's. Like many people caring for a loved one with dementia, we found ourselves swimming in questions. We began by gathering our family together to discuss their care options. Then, the years ahead taught us about the dos and don'ts of dementia care. It is my hope that you will benefit from reading the stories of my experiences as I cared for my loving parents.

As you read my stories, you might begin to feel that caregiving looks utterly overwhelming. I'll tell you there are times when it will feel that way. Indeed, there will be days of tears but also moments of laughter through tears. Along the way, I encourage you to embrace the everyday moments of simply holding your mom's hand and smiling into her face and telling her how much you love her, even if she can't find the words to tell you the same. Trust me, she hears you and she knows you are there.

Whenever possible, we engage our children in creative ways to show love for Mom and even other residents at her memory care. Something beautiful happens when you bring together children and seniors! As you create new memories with your mom, you will find that one day those joyful moments will far overshadow the challenges you faced.

While our family certainly endured the sadness that comes with the gradual fading of a lifetime of memories, we intentionally focused on celebrating the life that was still inside each of them. Our family will always hold dear the vivid memories of our mom and dad laughing and playing with their grandchildren, taking trips to the mountains with their adult children and grandchildren, and the two of them snuggling together, reading aloud the love letters they had written to one another more than 65 years prior.

During the years that I helped care for my parents, it was a longing of mine to teach my children that all human life holds immense value. I personally believe that a human's worth, at every stage, is intrinsic because it derives from God, who made human beings in his own image. My boys spent many years of their young lives helping to care for their Nana and Pop. I am truly thankful that the love they shared with their grandparents will be forever a part of them.

Making Watercolor Memories

Six months after my dad was diagnosed with early stage Alzheimer's, our family focused on creating special memories together. I deeply desired for my children to have a close bond with their grandparents. One crisp October day, Nana and Pop, along with my two boys (ages four and five) and I enjoyed a magical time together painting watercolor "leaves," while we laughed and shared stories. We collected an assortment of fall leaves from the yard and traced them onto water color paper. Each of us created our own unique masterpiece. Today those painted leaves are among my prize treasures. So, don't worry if you aren't an artistic person. You'd be amazed at the art inside of you and especially hidden inside the person with dementia! Art is a wonderful therapy.

—Halle

Dedications

Thank you

for your Inspiration, Guidance, Friendship, Motivation, and Encouragement.

Royanne Galas	Joseph Galas
Tim Dierks	Kenneth Hudak
Teepa Snow	P.K. Beville
Rodney Henderson	Eric Hadley
Tara Boyette	Lori Newcomb
Wendy Shoemaker	Pam Van Ahn
Paul Suggs	Sarah Maria Pieri
Michael Patterson	William Barbin
Cliff Smith	Teri Smith

The St Ives Memory Care Team

Abby Owolabi

Joseph Masini

Claribel Dupigny

Shunkelia Johnson

Melissa Morris

Susan F. Gale

—Keith Galas

To Mom.

I love you. I miss you every day.
You brought laughter and love to others,
even on your darkest days.
So blessed to be your daughter.

To Dad.

I love you.
You lived life to give yourself for others.
So thankful I can care for you now.

II Cor. 4:18

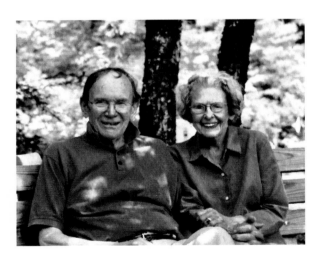

—Halle Eskew

Chapters

1

What do I
do now?

Dementia usually steps into people's lives in a subtle way. Typically, a family member will hear someone comment that their Mom seems to be forgetting things. Then Mom leaves the stove on or asks you to come over to help with the phone when it's really the remote. You start to worry. You take Mom to her regular doctor's appointment. Mom doesn't seem like herself and the doctor is concerned. The doctor recommends that Mom see a neurologist. Then you get the call that Mom has been diagnosed with Alzheimer's. You go to Mom and tell her that everything will be alright. You hold back tears because you need to be strong for her right now. You may feel like screaming, "Somebody help me!" So many questions race through your mind; What is Alzheimer's? Will Mom be safe in her house? Do I need to start looking for an assisted living facility? What type of paperwork should I start gathering? Will my family help me? Will Mom get worse?

The first priority is to make sure Mom knows she is loved and will be safe. The second priority is to get organized and to build a game plan. Compile notes about Mom's medical condition and find out if there are any legal or financial issues pending. Start to gather contact numbers, insurance information, account numbers and other important details. Gather any existing advanced directives, doctor information and paperwork specific to Mom's care.

There are several worksheets near the back of this book, including an organizational worksheet that can be used to create your own personal binder. These documents are also available as PDF downloads at www.parentaldementia.com.

This organizational worksheet is meant to help you navigate through the responsibilities you now must undertake. Please print or copy the worksheets and follow along.

Family Duties - Gather family and friends for a meeting to determine which roles each person will take in helping with Mom's care. Meet in person, by phone or by video chat. Discuss your goals, air feelings and divide up duties. Appoint a proxy to summarize the decisions made and distribute notes after the meeting. Start to build a file with the notes, medications, doctor information, value graph, visit schedule and a copy of the filled out "worksheet".

Try to distribute a copy of this file to everyone in the meeting. Also, be sure to include Mom in the decision-making process as well. If a power of attorney (POA) is already is in place, write down the family members that will be responsible for the health decisions and the financial decisions. Advanced Directives will be explained later.

Visits – If Mom is alone or starting to experience unsafe behavior, a visitation schedule will need to be arranged. Have family members agree to visit Mom at different times and days. Mom may need 24-hour supervision or just a few hours a day. Sometimes Mom may just need some company around in the late evening hours or just someone to help her take a walk. If Mom starts to wander around outside and gets lost in the neighborhood, a full day and night schedule may need to be created for a professional caregiver with dementia experience.

Medications – Assign someone to manage Mom's medications. This person will be responsible for arranging, administering and ordering Mom's medications as well as have a working knowledge of Mom's health issues. Medication will need to change as Mom's symptoms evolve. This person will also need to build a relationship with Mom's doctors and pharmacist and should be assigned to transport and accompany Mom to her medical appointments. In my experience, medication errors are a major cause of many terrible situations. Falls, confusion and agitation can all be caused by skipped meds or meds taken at the wrong time. Make a list of Mom's medications, including her self-care meds, and include it in the package to be given to everyone concerned. This list will also be useful for doctor's appointments. The responsible person should be the one to pick up the meds from the pharmacy. The pharmacist may have some concerns and need to speak to someone who knows your Mom's condition. This communication can help resolve medication errors and errors in the future.

Emergency Calls – Two people need to be assigned to be called in case of an emergency. The first person should be the POA in charge of health decisions and the second person should be someone who is both reliable and easy to reach.

Care – Have a discussion about your Mom's care options. (These options will be explained thoroughly in an upcoming chapter named "What are my options?")

Doctors – Make a list of all of Mom's doctors. Gather the doctor's name, address, and phone number, the office nurse's name and the doctor's specialty. (neurologist, oncologist, dentist, general physician.) Also, include any VA information.

Hair – I have found that your Mom's hair salon is going to be important for a while. (Same for Dad's barbershop) The hair salon is where Mom can feel like a woman. Assign the person that understands this to oversee scheduling these appointments and transporting Mom to the salon.

Food – Is Mom eating? Is Mom losing weight? This can be caused by many issues. Mom may feel insecure about using the oven and too embarrassed to ask for help. Mom may not like to eat alone or simply forgets to eat. Assign someone to help make meals and eat together with Mom. Sometimes Mom will forget the purpose of utensils and may need some encouragement to get started. Studies have shown that finger foods are better for people with higher acuity dementia.[1]

ICD (Pacemaker) - Assign someone to monitor the pacemaker. The ICD should be checked regularly to find out how the wires are working, how the battery is doing, and how Mom's condition and any external devices have affected the ICD's performance. Mom's doctor may check her ICD several times a year by office visit, over the phone or through an Internet connection. An ICD's batteries will last typically four to seven years.

Advance Directives - Advance care planning involves learning about the types of decisions that might need to be made, considering those decisions ahead of time, and then letting others know about Mom's preferences. These preferences are often put into an advance directive, a legal document that goes into effect only if Mom is unable to speak for herself. This could be the result of a disease like dementia. It helps others know what type of medical care Mom will want. It also allows Mom to express her values and desires related to end-of-life care. Sometimes when doctors believe a cure is no longer possible, decisions must be made about the use of emergency treatments to keep Mom alive.

For a free printable advance directive, visit the AARP website.

https://www.aarp.org/caregiving/financial-legal/
free-printable-advance-directives/?intcmp=AE-CAR-LEG-R3-C1-LL2

Living will - A living will is a document in which you can stipulate the kind of life-prolonging medical care you want if you become terminally ill, permanently unconscious, or in a vegetative state and unable to make your own decisions. Many states have their own living-will forms, each with somewhat different requirements.

POA - Power of attorney is granted to an attorney-in-fact or agent to give that individual the legal authority to make decisions for an incapacitated principal. The laws for creating a power of attorney vary from state to state, but there are certain general guidelines to follow. Before you or a loved one signs any documents, however, be sure to consult with an attorney concerning all applicable laws and regulations.

The principal determines the amount of power given to the POA, and this individual can be given the authority to deal with only one particular issue (a Specific power of attorney), or to handle most of the principal's personal and financial matters (a General power of attorney). Regardless of the type of power of attorney granted, the POA is responsible for keeping accurate records of all transactions that he or she makes on behalf of the principal. The POA also is responsible for distinguishing between the types of decisions he or she has the power to make and those the POA cannot make. 2

There are multiple types of decisions that the POA can be given the power to make.

- Making financial decisions
- Recommending a guardian
- Making health care decisions, including the ability to consent to giving, withholding, or stopping medical treatments, services, or diagnostic procedures.

(Note: your loved one can also make a separate "health care power of attorney" to give only this power to an individual)

DNR – Do-not-resuscitate (DNR) is a legal order written to withhold cardio-pulmonary resuscitation (CPR) or advanced cardiac life support (ACLS), in respect of the wishes of a patient in case their heart was to stop or they were to stop breathing. A DNR may also be called a no code or allow natural death order. The DNR request is usually made by the patient or a health care power of attorney and allows the medical teams taking care of the patient to respect their wishes. A DNR does not affect any treatment other than that which would require intubation or CPR. Patients who are DNR can continue to get chemotherapy, antibiotics, dialysis, or any other appropriate treatments.

POLST / MOLST – A number of states use an advance care planning form known as POLST (Physician Orders for Life-Sustaining Treatment) or MOLST (Medical Orders for Life-Sustaining Treatment). This form provides more detailed guidance about your medical care preferences.

The form is filled out by your doctor, or sometimes a nurse practitioner or physician's assistant, after discussing your wishes with you and your family. Once signed by your doctor, this form has the same authority as any other medical order. Check with your state department of health to find out if this form is available where you live.

Donation –Over 125 million people are registered as organ donors, but only about three in 1,000 or .003 percent can become donors when they die. The process of donation most often begins with your consent to be a donor by registering in your state. Anyone, regardless of age or medical history, can sign up to be a donor. A transplant team will determine at an individual's time of death whether a donation is possible. There's no age limit to organ donation. To date, the oldest donor in the U.S. was age 93. What matters is the health and condition of your organs at the time of death.[3]

To find out more about organ donation, visit www.organdonor.gov.

Values – Mom likely doesn't want to think about her final days, but planning for them now is helpful to those who love and care for her. It also helps make sure that you will know and respect her wishes. If you are unsure of Mom's wishes, some insightful questions will help clear this up. Mom may have strong opinions about what is important to her at the very end of life. She may want certain things she dislikes to be avoided. You may know your mom better than anyone, but asking questions early enough about her values and beliefs can help you with some difficult decisions that may need to be made. I have added a chart to help you with asking these questions. The best way to go through these questions is to ask, "How important is it to you... "then ask the question. Some of these questions are delicate and may upset your mom. Be mindful of her feelings while asking these intimate questions. Take your time and try to have a conversation as you go along.

Print Value Question PDF at www.parentaldementia.com

Caregiver Interviews

If the decision is to keep Mom at home and to bring in an outside caregiver, I strongly suggest that you seek out referrals. You might find someone in your area that has used an independent caregiver or a home care company that they can recommend. There are some helpful online neighborhood apps that offer a great way to reach out to families in your situation who may live nearby. You may even decide to organize a support group with other people who share a mutual need for encouragement and who are willing to share their experiences. Finding the right caregiver and the right home care company is more an art than a science. Once you've got your contacts, I strongly suggest interviewing a few candidates before signing paperwork. Ask open ended questions, such as, what do you like most about being a caregiver?

Ask the caregiver their thoughts on your mom's care. Get them to tell stories about their past clients. Ask what they would do in certain situations. Keep in mind you have every right to be hesitant about a stranger in your home, just as the candidate is apprehensive about you. Always remember that the caregiver can say no to your mom as you can say no to their care. When the caregivers are chosen, write down their names and contact information on the worksheet. Some agencies will not allow their caregivers to share their personal phone numbers.

Please review the 20 questions to ask potential care providers - provided by Comfort Keepers at www.parentaldementia.com

Home Care Interviews

Home care companies have access to many types of caregivers. Some home care companies only have five to 10 caregivers and other larger home care companies could have over 200 caregivers on their roster. They may offer male or female, young or more mature. Most importantly, they may have caregivers with dementia care experience.

Home care companies are responsible for the caregivers criminal background check, TB test and drug test. Also, most home care companies offer yearly state mandatory training to their caregivers. When you find two to three companies that you feel can offer good caregivers for your mom write down the company names and contact information on the "worksheet".

Notes on Home Care: The biggest benefit to home care is that Mom can stay at home. Mom will not have to transition into a new environment. Although you must also consider that Mom will now have a stranger in her home. This is a transition in itself. Mom may push back and not like the caregiver and tell you to fire the caregiver or she may love the caregiver and treat her as a new member of the family.

Budget can also be a factor. The cost for an experienced caregiver from a home care company will typically be around $19.00 to $22.00 an hour with a four to eight hour minimum shift. (Time and a half on holidays) Also, be prepared for call offs, vacations and sick days from your caregiver. A quality home care company will be able to replace your caregiver in a few hours. Although, the replacement may not know your mother's daily routine which could cause some agitation. Try to work with an established home care company if possible. They will be more willing and able to handle these types of issues when they pop up.

Community Tours

When deciding on a memory care community, once again, consider getting solid referrals which are typically found by word of mouth. Don't be afraid to bring up your situation when talking to friends. You will be surprised at how willing people are to recommend a community that they have experience with or have heard about. Call at least four to five communities and ask to speak to someone concerning your mother.

You typically will speak with the marketing director or the executive director. Explain your situation to them and discuss your mother's needs. Try to narrow down your search to two or three communities and then schedule a tour. A tour will typically take about an hour.

Print out a few copies of my Tour Checklist at www.parentaldementia.com to help guide you on what to ask and what to keep your eyes on. When you choose the communities to tour, write down their names and contact information on the worksheet. (Also found at www.parentaldementia.com)

Referral Services

Referral services are designed to guide and suggest communities in your desired location that fit your mother's needs. These companies should offer you a detailed report that includes information on age of building, prices, resident capacity, care type, survey scores and overall reputation.

So that families won't have to pay for this service, communities sign contracts with referral sources and agree to pay a percentage of the first month's bill (combining rent and care). Keep in mind that not all communities use these services and if you agree to have a service help you hunt for the best community for your mom, they may not recommend the communities without a contract with the referral service.

With that being said, referral services, especially in large cities, have become very helpful in this process. Seek out an agent that is truly familiar with the city where you are located. There are many remarkable service agents that can help you through this difficult learning process.

Many agents will offer to tour with you and help you through this process face-to-face, whereas other agents may offer quality assistance but you will never meet in person.

Write down the referral service's agents name and contact information on the "worksheet".

Insurance

There are many types of insurance. Keep the insurance information with this worksheet. There is health insurance, Medicare, Medicaid, long-term care insurance, and veterans insurance. Veterans Affairs offers a benefit that is called Aid and Attendance. This benefit is extremely helpful to many veterans' families, including the veteran themselves, the surviving spouse, the married couple and even the surviving spouse with dependent. (Refer to chapter 13 for more information on financial options.)

For more information on the VA benefit visit www.veteranaid.org/apply.php

Hospital of Choice

We can all agree that some hospitals are better than others. If Mom has a fall and needs to go to the hospital, sometimes the ambulance will make the decision which hospital to take her to for her care. This decision is not always made in Mom's best interest. If you or your mom feels strongly about a hospital, please share this feeling with the emergency personnel and demand the ambulance take her to your hospital of choice. You must advocate for your mom's care at all times especially at the hospital where nurses are often overloaded with patients. Due to the confusion and sometimes communication challenges that accompany dementia, Mom may need additional care and attention.

You know your mom best and can be her voice. If you can't be at the hospital, it may be necessary to hire a caregiver to provide another layer of care through the night. This will be an added expense to her hospital stay.

AMBULANCE DISPATCH

At around 8 p.m. one evening, I received a call from my Resident Care Director. She informed me that a resident had a bad fall and needed to go to the hospital. She confirmed that family was called and told of the incident and would be meeting their mom at the hospital. The ambulance arrived and agreed to take our resident to the family's hospital of choice. At around 10 p.m. I received another call from my resident care director telling me that the family called and was very upset because their mother never showed up at the hospital. I told the nurse to call 911 and ask where they took our resident and I would start calling all the area hospital emergency rooms. I called four hospital ERs and was told that the woman was not there.

I then received a call back from my nurse who said that 911 confirmed that the ambulance was re-routed to a different hospital by the ambulance dispatch. So I called back that hospital again to ask about our resident. To my surprise, the ER front desk said that they had no woman there by that name. I explained that the 911 dispatch told us that they took our resident to this hospital. It was now 11:45 p.m. and this lady was yelling at me, "She is not here ... what do you not understand, Sir?" I asked her to please look one more time. She responded, "I have looked on the white board, and there is no .... hold please!"

I held for 10 minutes, "Sir ... found your lady. She is waiting to see the doctor. Did you know that she has dementia?" I then called my nurse, who then called the family and explained everything at about 12 a.m.. My resident was back in the community at 3 a.m. and her family was very tired and frustrated.

An ambulance EMT may have no control over which hospital they deliver to and sometimes they are actualy re-routed to a totally different city. The last thing dispatch is worried about is calling the community with this new information.

−Keith

Hospitals: Overworked and Understaffed Nurses

My mom had mid-stage Alzheimer's when she became severely lethargic and unable to walk. She was rushed to a nearby hospital (one our family had previously deemed to be a solid medical facility.) The doctors were quick to diagnose my mom with pneumonia and began treating her. After two days, I saw her reaching for her lower right side and moaning.

I knew there was something terribly wrong and I thought she had possibly been misdiagnosed. I asked the head nurse to order a CT scan right away.

Surprisingly, the nurses were reluctant to explore my mom's condition any further and dismissed her pain as a case of gas in her abdomen. I began to realize that there was a shortage of nurses on the floor and perhaps they were simply eager to move on to the next person in their long line of patients. I came in the next day and found they had done an x-ray, not a CT scan. The nurse believed the x-ray confirmed her gas pain. I did not agree. My mom was on day three of moaning and holding her side. I made a quick call to the hospital director to insist that she receive a CT scan immediately. The hospital complied. Results showed that she did not have pneumonia at all but instead was suffering from a gangrenous gallbladder. The doctor ordered emergency surgery to remove her gallbladder.

One year later, my mom was taken to the same hospital by ambulance after falling at her community. Sadly, we discovered the nursing staff was even more sparse and negligent than before. We never allowed my mom to be taken to that hospital again. The next hospital we chose was across town, but the nursing staff was amazing!

My advice: Choose the best hospital, not the one that is the most convenient.

–Halle

Budgets

Calculate the budget for each form of care for your mom. This will help when discussing the options with your family. Unless money is not an issue, the question will typically be: How much is this going to cost? Calculate a typical month for each choice.

For example: Home care 8 hrs @ $19 = $152.00

M-F is 5 x $152.00 = $760 a week / $3,040 a month + living expenses

So in this scenario you would write: Home care $3,040.00 + Home and Food

Day care is typically a set fee for the day that includes a breakfast and lunch. Sometimes day care companies will also include or provide transportation for a small fee. If Mom needs additional care they may also need to include an up charge for meds, incontinence or redirection. Day care is typically Monday through Friday and hours are around 8 a.m. to 6 p.m.

Let's say Mom is going to move in with your family and go to day care five days week.

20 days @ $145 a day = $2,900.00 a month

So in this scenario you would write: Day care $2,900.00 + Home and Food

2

What is Dementia?

Dementia is a group of symptoms that affects cognitive tasks such as memory and reasoning. Think of the term dementia as an umbrella that covers a group of symptoms affecting memory, thinking, and social abilities severely enough to interfere with daily functioning. Dementia is caused by damage to brain cells. This damage interferes with the ability of brain cells to communicate with each other. When brain cells cannot communicate effectively, thinking, behavior and feelings can be affected. Tens of millions of people worldwide experience dementia today. It is reasonable to assume that Alzheimer's could affect as much as 75 million by 2030 and over 130 million by 2050. Many of those affected will likely be in developing countries. Over 50 percent of people with dementia now live in low and middle-income countries, and the occurrence is increasing.[1] It is expected that for those living past age 55, one in six women, and one in 10 men will develop dementia during their lifetime.[2]

The most common types of dementia include:

Alzheimer's

Alzheimer's disease is among the leading causes of death in the United States. While deaths from other major diseases have declined significantly in recent years, deaths from Alzheimer's are on the rise, with a 120 percent jump from 2000 to 2018.

Symptoms: Difficulty remembering recent conversations, names or events is often an early clinical symptom; apathy and depression are also often early symptoms. Later symptoms include impaired communication, poor judgment, disorientation, confusion, behavior changes and difficulty speaking, swallowing and walking.[3]

Vascular dementia

Previously known as multi-infarct or post-stroke dementia, vascular dementia is less common as a sole cause of dementia than Alzheimer's, accounting for about 10 percent of dementia cases. Blood vessel blockage, damage leading to infarcts (strokes), and bleeding in the brain are all considered vascular dementia.

Symptoms: Impaired judgment or ability to make decisions, plan or organize is more likely to be the initial symptom.[4]

Lewy bodies (LBD)

Lewy body dementia is the most common category of progressive dementia other than Alzheimer's disease dementia. Lewy bodies are protein deposits that develop in brain cells involved in thinking, memory, and movement.

Symptoms: People with Lewy bodies often have memory loss and thinking problems common in Alzheimer's, but are more likely than people with Alzheimer's to have initial or early symptoms such as sleep disturbances, well-formed visual hallucinations, slowness, gait imbalance or other Parkinson like movement features.[5]

Parkinson's disease

Parkinson's disease is a neurodegenerative disorder that primarily affects the dopamine producing neurons in the part of the brain known as the substantial nigra. As Parkinson's disease progresses, it often results in a dementia similar to Lewy bodies or Alzheimer's.[6]

Symptoms: Symptoms begin appearing between the ages of 50 and 60. They develop slowly and often go unnoticed by family, friends, and even the person who has them. The progression of symptoms often varies from one person to another due to the diversity of the disease. People with Parkinson's may experience tremors, mainly at rest. Also, changes in speech, slowness of movement, gait and balance issues and physical stiffness may occur.[7]

Frontotemporal dementia

FTD is similar to Alzheimer's in that it also causes progressive, irreversible degeneration of brain cells.

Symptoms: Typical symptoms include changes in personality and behavior and difficulty with language. Nerve cells in the front and side regions of the brain are especially affected.[8]

Creutzfeldt-Jakob disease

CJD is the most common human form of a group of rare, fatal brain disorders affecting people and certain other mammals. Variant CJD (mad cow disease) occurs most often in cattle, and has been transmitted to people under certain circumstances. As of 2016, 231 cases of CJD have been reported worldwide.

Symptoms: Rapidly fatal disorder that impairs memory and coordination and causes behavior changes.[9]

Huntington's disease

Huntington's disease is a brain disorder that is progressive. It is initiated by a single defective gene on chromosome four.

Symptoms: Abnormal involuntary movements, decline in thinking and reasoning skills, and irritability, depression and other mood changes.[10]

Korsakoff Syndrome

Korsakoff syndrome is a persistent brain disorder affecting memory that is caused by severe deficiency of thiamine (vitamin B-1). The most common cause is alcohol abuse.

Symptoms: Memory problems may be strikingly severe while other thinking and social skills seem relatively unaffected.[11]

Mixed dementia

In mixed dementia, abnormalities linked to more than one cause of dementia occur concurrently in the brain. Recent studies suggest that mixed dementia is more common than previously thought.

https://www.alz.org/media/Documents/alzheimers-dementia-mixed-dementia-ts.pdf

3

How do I know if Mom is getting Dementia?

The Sneaky First Signs of Dementia

Dad was 76 years old when our family first saw his signs of dementia. My dad and I were driving home from a family beach trip at the Florida Gulf Coast when he asked a simple question, *"When will Gary (my brother) arrive in town?"* Dad asked that same question, perhaps four times more, in less than an hour. Each time he asked the question, it was as if it was the first time. Like coastal waves washing over his words, his thoughts were erased in a rush of water. My heart was flooded with sadness and I knew I needed to reach out to his friends to see if there were other signs of memory loss. Stories emerged of missed lunch appointments and other mishaps. A follow up appointment to the neurologist determined that he had cognitive impairment related to Alzheimer's. The doctor then prescribed medications to help slow down the disease's progression. These signs were a warning call to start planning for his future care. Thankfully, we did. Within a few years he was struggling to manage his finances and reason through difficult decisions. We already had a plan in place that helped to prevent further problems. If you see signs in Mom that concern you, don't be afraid to investigate further.

–Halle

The early signs of dementia may not be immediately obvious. If your mom has several of the below warning signs of dementia, consult a doctor for a complete assessment.

Short term memory issues - Mom may be able to remember events that took place years ago but not what she had for lunch. Short-term memory also includes frequently losing things, struggling to remember why she entered a particular room, or forgetting what she was supposed to do on any given day.

Difficulty in completing tasks - This usually starts with Mom having difficulty doing more complex tasks like balancing a checkbook or playing games that have a lot of rules.

Difficulty following storylines - Just as finding and using the right words becomes difficult, Mom may forget the meanings of words or struggle to follow along with conversations or TV programs.

Communication issues – Mom may have difficulty explaining something or finding the right words to express her thoughts. Sometimes having a conversation with someone that has early dementia can be difficult, and it may take patience. Let Mom work through her wording and try not to show any facial frustration.

Mood and Personality issues - It isn't always easy to recognize this, but you may notice a change in Mom's moods when it comes to family members or friends. Mom may snap at a granddaughter or be upset with a friend for no apparent reason.

Along with mood changes, you might also see a shift in personality. One typical example of personality change seen with dementia is a shift from being shy to outgoing. This is because the disease often affects judgment.

Apathy issues – Mom could lose interest in hobbies or activities. She may lose interest in spending time with friends and family. You may notice a general *laissez faire* attitude. This can be a dangerous time for Mom. This may be the time when Mom suspects something is wrong and may become severely depressed. Be aware of this issue as a possible warning sign for suicide.

Confusion - Confusion may arise as Mom can no longer recognize faces or find the right words, or if she struggles to interact socially with friends.

Failing sense of direction - The sense of direction and spatial orientation commonly starts to worsen with the onset of dementia. Mom may not recognize once familiar landmarks and forget regularly used directions. It also becomes more difficult to follow step-by-step instructions, such as for recipes and medications.

Repetitive - Mom may repeat daily tasks, such as checking the mail or she may gather items obsessively. You may notice that the hair brush is in the refrigerator or the bedroom pillows are all in the bathroom. She may repeat the same questions.

Adapt to change – Mom may forget why she went to the store and get lost on the way home. She will find comfort in routine and may avoid trying new experiences. Mom may become more likely to make excuses to stay home rather than go to church or visit a friend.

The twists and turns of dementia

Within five years after my dad's Alzheimer's diagnosis, my mom began to exhibit signs of dementia in her early 80's. While his cognitive loss had exhibited itself in a severe decline of memory and reasoning, my mom's disease manifestation was uniquely different. Since both my parents were living with my family, I could observe their day-to-day habits. One afternoon, I discovered a clear plastic bag filled with dozens of tops from all my mom's toothpaste tubes and other toiletry items. Apparently, she had saved the assorted tops because she was struggling to return them to their rightful place. It appeared that her executive function was slipping away. Another loss arrived as her once beautiful handwriting and flawless spelling skills began fading away. She had been an elementary school teacher and possessed beautiful penmanship. I found grocery lists with half written words that drifted off the page.

Perhaps the most confusing sign was her loss of vision. Although she had undergone cataract surgery on both her eyes and tested out with 20/30 vision, she would often say she couldn't see. I took her to several doctors but no problem could be found. It was a couple of years before I understood that it was actually her brain that couldn't see, not her eyes. It broke my heart that she had lost her vision. She was an artist and had loved to look at pretty things. It became clear that day that the tangles of the Alzheimer's brain forge a uniquely different path in each person who struggles with this type of dementia.

—Halle

4

What is Sundowning?

Sundowning is a neurological phenomenon associated with increased confusion and restlessness. It's also known as late-day confusion. Approximately 20% of people with dementia suffer from some degree of Sundowning. Mom's confusion and agitation may get worse in the late afternoon and evening. Agitation can be brought on by many conditions and/or situations. Some medical professionals believe that Sundowning is an accumulation of all of the sensory stimulation from the day that becomes overwhelming and causes stress. Others speculate that it is caused by hormonal imbalances that occur at night. Another theory suggests that the onset of symptoms at night is simply due to fatigue, while even others believe it has to do with the anxiety caused by the inability to see as well in the dark. Experienced behaviorists argue that lack of sleep, hunger, thirst, pain and loneliness can also bring on this neurological phenomenon also.[12]

After all my research, I believe that the "expert findings" on why Sundowning occurs with dementia is somewhat unclear. In my experience, the most common trigger of Sundowning is negative or stressful situations. Mom may be reliving a stressful moment in her normal routine from 30 years ago. For example, Mom may be concerned that her husband is coming home and dinner won't be ready in time. Do not respond: "Mom, don't you know that Dad passed away three years ago?" This will elevate the confusion and the agitation. A better response would be "It's alright Mom. Dinner will be ready soon. Let's go wash our hands and get ready." This will give you the opportunity to have a conversation and change the subject, which will defuse her agitation. If Mom is constantly corrected, it could trigger her agitation and continue to elevate her Sundowning throughout the evening.

Always remember, to your Mom this situation is her reality. Therefore, telling her that she is wrong is not helping her. It's not always important to be right or for Mom to be right. *"Just go with it."*

The Art of Redirection

When I train my team of caregivers on redirection, I ask them to imagine themselves in a scenario in which it is in everyone's best interest to switch the focus of attention to boost the mood to a happier tone. For example, imagine sitting in the passenger seat of their car waiting to go out to dinner with someone special. I ask them to think about the restaurant that they will be going to and how excited they are to spend time with their date. I ask them to imagine that their date gets in the driver's seat in a bad mood and starts griping about the kids or the neighbor's lawn. I ask them to imagine that they change the subject with something like: "Hey, look at that truck... I bet you would look good in a truck like that!" or "Why don't we stop by DQ on the way home so we can split a sundae?"

I ask my caregivers if they have ever done something like that. I bet around 90 percent of them say, "Yes, all the time." I then ask them to role play and redirect a common situation during Sundowning.

These responses sometimes take a little practice and knowledge of likes and dislikes. But just like it is more important to have a nice date than get upset about a negative situation adding fuel to the fire, it is more important to *"just go with it"* rather than to draw even more attention to am upsetting topic and elevate Mom's agitation.

A common Sundowning agitation is when Mom doesn't know what time it is and what she is supposed to be doing at that specific moment. This can be reduced by keeping a routine for bedtime. Have dinner, pajamas and hygiene routines at the same time and keep a nightlight on in the bedroom to help reduce agitation when surroundings are unfamiliar.

Plan activities throughout the day and discourage long daytime naps. Try to switch Mom to decaf or keep caffeinated drinks for the morning and early afternoon only. Try to keep violent movies and crime shows off the TV at night. These visions will sometimes become Mom's reality and nighttime wondering and hallucinations could follow. Familiar music can also help to transition Mom to a happy place. When playing music, make sure you only play her favorite songs; unfamiliar songs may cause agitation and confusion.

When we don't know a resident's favorite songs, I have found that piano music or soft jazz works best in the late evenings.

Medications - Often, medications are needed to minimize problems related to Sundowning.

The common medications that are used to manage evening agitation and behavioral disturbances associated with Sundowning are benzodiazepines, such as Xanax, Valium, Ativan and Restoril which can reduce anxiety and promote sleep. Antipsychotics, such as haloperidol (Haldol) and droperidol are also prescribed. Aricept, Exelon, and Razadyne are often used to help memory issues.

The Backyard Christmas Play

My young boys and their friends excitedly put together costumes and props for a backyard Christmas play. The play was scheduled to start at 8pm so it would be dark enough to use spotlights. My mom had been full of anticipation about the children's performance. Later that evening, I went to her room to call her for the start of the show. When I looked into her face to tell her it was time to go, I encountered a completely different person. Instead of her usual light-hearted demeanor, I discovered someone who was irritated and upset. She refused to go outside to watch the play. My heart sank. I didn't know what was happening as I had never seen her this way before. I tried to reason with her but she was adamant.

I later realized that she had been sundowning. The next morning, she was her usual cheerful self and ready to play with the boys. From then on I began to look for signs of sundowning and sought ways to redirect my mom and dad if they were feeling restless or disoriented.

–Halle

5

Why is everyone telling me to get help?

A family member that is caring for Mom with dementia, often called the invisible second patient, is 20 times more likely to be depressed than if Mom had a physical disability. The effects of being a family caregiver, though sometimes a positive experience, are generally negative, with high rates of burn out, psychological issues as well as social isolation.

Caregivers face many obstacles as they balance caregiving with other demands, including child rearing, career, and relationships. They are at an increased risk for stress, depression, and a variety of other health complications. Caregivers tend to be so focused on their loved one that they don't realize their own health and well-being are suffering. The effects on caregivers can be complex. There are many other factors that may exacerbate how caregivers react and feel as a result of their role. Studies on dementia caregivers found that nearly 25 percent provided 40 plus hours of care per week (compared with 15 percent for non-dementia caregivers). This included personal care such as bathing, feeding, and assisting with toileting for 65 percent of caregivers. More than 70 percent of caregivers sustained this commitment for more than one year and only 30 percent for four or more years.

If you are a caregiver and are feeling overwhelmed or constantly worried, you are not alone.

It may be time for you to take a break in your caregiving. Other warning signs are feeling tired all the time, unusually irritated, weight issues, losing interest in activities you used to enjoy, having frequent headaches, or an overall sadness. Sometimes a caregiver will turn to alcohol and drugs. If this describes you, it is time for a break from your mom's care. You need to reevaluate your priorities and take some *me time*. Unfortunately, mom's dementia will still be there when you get back.

Hand off your mom's care to another family member or hire a professional live-in caregiver if possible.[13] The bad news is that you will instantly feel guilty that you somehow failed your mom and you will think that no one will be able to do the job as well as you because you are the only one that understands your mom. The good news is that after a few days of not feeling the pressure of caregiving, you will eventually exhale and start to look at your own life again with renewed energy. You may even start thinking of what makes you happy. You may actually be amazed that someone can look after your mom and the world did not end. The sun came up, birds are singing and Mom will be okay today. I am not saying that anyone could ever love your mom more than you, I am just explaining that if you don't take care of yourself, your body will quit on you and your family will be making plans for your care as well. If you're on a plane and the oxygen masks drop down, they tell you to take care of yourself first before you can help anyone else.

The Guilt Trap

When my dad was diagnosed with Alzheimer's, I knew immediately I wanted to help care for him. He spent his whole life caring for our family and he was always trying to help and serve others who were in need. Caring for others was at the core of his being. His genuine desire to help others was born out of his personal relationship with Christ. The decision to have my parents move from Alabama to live with our family felt right. We reasoned that it was an opportunity for them to be near some of their grandchildren and close by so we could more easily care for them in their aging years.

Mom and Dad lived with us for nearly five years, before we realized that it was time for everyone to make a change. While those years were filled with sweet memories, I found that I was feeling increasingly depressed and isolated. Most importantly, we knew that my parents were no longer safe at home alone during the times when we needed to leave the house. And, home care was no longer an option as my dad began to resent caregivers coming to the house. The final event that led us to find a memory care community for my parents was my mom's gallbladder surgery. The anesthesia from surgery had affected her cognitive function and overall mood. We knew it was time to seek out social interaction and safer surroundings. Even still, I felt guilty on every side! It seemed that I was choosing between my health and that of my parents. There appeared to be no good choices. Thankfully, I was wrong. While there were challenges in transitioning them into a memory care community (I'll share that story in Chapter 12), we soon realized this new season was best for everyone.

Our family visited Mom and Dad in their residence twice a week. The boys started putting on magic shows and plays for all the residents. Slowly, my guilt evaporated. I became stronger and finally able to be a better wife, mom, daughter and friend.

–Halle

6

What are my options?

Families tend to first try to keep Mom in her home where there will be little to no change in environment and therefore very little confusion. This decision is typically aligned with the wishes of Mom and other family members. When I hear from a son or daughter that it's a "family decision", I know that it usually means that they will try to keep Mom at home as long as possible or until an event occurs. An *event* can be a small issue like flooding the bathroom floor or calling the police because of a hallucination to possibly something very bad resulting in injury, hospitalization and sometimes surgery. I receive emails weekly from families and referral sources reporting sad news about a potential resident that may have stayed in their home too long.

Option 1 is usually to keep Mom at home with the occasional *drop-in* from family members. When Mom needs more help, you may hire a caregiver to stay with Mom. Then in time, two caregivers spread throughout the day, 7 days a week.

Option 2 is adult day care, where Mom spends a few days a week at day care and maybe with a caregiver a few nights a week at home. This may change to 5 days a week at an adult day care and a family member picks Mom up and spends the night over at Mom's house and then redirects her throughout the night. On weekends, when the day care is closed, another family member comes in and stays with Mom. Obviously, this continued option can be stressful on the family.

Option 3 is providing a space for Mom in a family member's home with additional help from a professional caregiver. This option can be great for a period of time. You must keep an eye out for possible isolation behaviors and the onset of depression.

Option 4 is memory care. This is where Mom will receive 24-hour supervised care. The 24-hour supervised care does not mean one-on-one care. It means that Mom will be in a safe environment with help nearby. Most memory care communities offer around an 8:1 care ratio, which means that one caregiver is responsible for eight residents. With care ratios, you must keep in mind that for most of the day Mom will be involved in group activities that require very little one on one attention. Group activities such as singing, bingo, watching a movie, and music entertainment usually are overseen by a qualified activity leader and also a caregiver to help assist with fall risk residents.

A combination of Option 1, Option 2 and Option 3 are also sometimes used.

Some people will say, "Hey, what about independent living or assisted living or continuing care retirement communities (CCRC) or adult family homes?" Well, none of those choices are typically a tremendous option for dementia care. As for a CCRC, Mom would have already made the decision to move into that type of situation long before she was diagnosed with dementia.

But, here is the scoop anyway:

Independent Living – Independent living communities offer dining services, basic housekeeping, transportation, activities, social programs, and access to exercise equipment. Many also offer emergency alert systems, live-in managers, and amenities like pools, spas, clubhouses, and on-site beauty and barber salons. Independent Living is a wonderful option for most seniors.

Dementia care is not offered and is typically a reason for management to present a 30-day notice of discharge. Often a couple will move to a beautiful independent community together and truly love it. Unfortunately, the husband or wife may develop mild dementia and the other spouse will attempt to be the caregiver. This situation can be manageable for a short period of time. From my experience, a heartbreaking relationship dynamic will start to occur.

First, the caregiving spouse will begin to notice that their friends are making excuses to not spend time with them. This will evolve into ignoring and eye rolling when in the dining room or participating in activities. The entire community will slowly move away from what they consider an "awkward" situation. There is occasionally that friend or couple that will always be there for help and support.

Assisted Living - Assisted living is geared more towards helping residents who need assistance with activities such as bathing, grooming, dressing, doing laundry and managing medications. Some AL communities will accommodate dementia residents as long as they are not exit-seeking and they are not experiencing Sundowning. These communities usually are not trained in redirection and dementia care. The activities are also not designed for dementia residents.

Continuing Care Retirement Communities (CCRC) - This option provides seniors the opportunity to live in one location for the duration of their life, with much of their future care already figured out.

Living in a community with multiple care options can take the stress out of the possible caregiving relationship and can create a great level of comfort for both Mom and the family. CCRC campuses are typically located in peaceful and welcoming surroundings. They are typically upscale communities set apart in choice locations that offer a great deal of privacy and convenience. Entry fees can run from around $20,000 up to over $1 million, with monthly charges ranging from $100 to over $5,000.

Adult Family Homes or Personal Care Homes are quite different from other types of senior care options in that they are generally limited to 6 to 10 residents at a time. Staffing is usually a couple caregivers and a full time LPN/RN. Adult family homes can be cozier than other larger senior living communities, which often resemble a hotel or resort.

However, adult family homes typically don't provide specific care for dementia or other specialized conditions. I have observed locations that have a caregiver with dementia training, but usually the property prefers to not admit dementia residents mainly because of the fear of elopement. (leaving the property unsupervised).

The monthly rental cost/care in an adult family home will vary greatly, depending on location, care and amenities. Monthly costs range from $2,800 to $6,700, with the average cost being around $4,000 per month nationally.

A Temporary Option is Respite Care - For the 60 million Americans caring for a loved one, respite care can serve a couple valuable functions. Respite is often used when a family caregiver needs to travel or just needs a break. Because of the high stress associated with caring for a loved one with dementia, respite care is a practical way to get a much needed "time out." Many memory care communities offer a 30-day respite as a test for a family to decide whether a community is right for them. The community will make a fully furnished model apartment their respite apartment or have a designated respite apartment ready to rent. Rates will vary across the country, but in my experience, respite rates range from $80 to $150 a day.

Possibly just a few hours to relax with others facing the same issues may be all you need to mentally recharge. In North Atlanta, there is a wonderful place that offers a unique day respite for caregivers and those with dementia. Amy's Place offers a way to socialize, play games, and just relax for a couple hours for free. These services are found in Europe, but extremely rare here in the United States. I pray similar places will pop up throughout America.

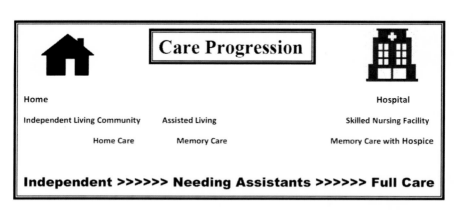

7

What is Home Care?

I f the decision has been made to take care of Mom in her home or have Mom move in with a family member, this scenario should be called step-up time. Basically, what this means is that a family member will step up and take responsibility for Mom's care. This will take a huge commitment. Often a family member will put his or her own life on pause. Family members have quit their jobs, moved to another state or even added on to their existing house. Many times I have been invited to a home to complete an assessment for entrance to my community and have seen remarkable attempts in keeping their mom as independent as possible. Families have moved to the second floor to give the living room as a secure area for their mom or added a studio apartment on to a house for Mom's safety and dignity. No one knows Mom better than her own family. This is important when understanding is needed.

When Mom has anxiety and needs love and reassurance, there is nobody better than her husband, daughter, son or close friend. With the right training, education and a lot of help, this scenario can work for a few good years. Although, when Mom becomes frustrated and acts out, hiring a professional caregiver can be extremely important to help prevent accidents. Unfortunately, the eventuality of Mom's care will generally take a turn, demanding alternative care options.

The top 5 reasons that cause families to look for alternatives to home care:

1) A Fall or Multiple Falls
2) Medication Confusion
3) Home Safety Issues
4) Caregiver Burnout
5) Hygiene Issues

---

1) A Fall or Multiple Falls

A heartbreaking event that unfortunately occurs is when Mom stumbles and falls.

Falls don't always occur because of balance issues. Falls can occur because of bone issues too. Has a friend ever told you that her Mom fell and broke her hip? I bet you have never heard a friend more accurately say, "My mom broke her hip and fell." If Mom falls and hurts herself, she will typically be sent to the hospital's emergency room. If there is no head injury, Mom will be observed and hopefully discharged. If there are broken bones or medical trauma your doctor may order a rehab visit that could last around 90 days (depending on insurance),

This is an ideal time to investigate other viable care options. If the decision is to have Mom back home, the section on Home Safety will be helpful.

2) Medication Confusion

Be prepared to manage medications. Most memory care residents are prescribed more than eight meds to be taken at precise times throughout the day. Some residents have moved into my community with over 20 meds and supplements that have been prescribed for them from three different doctors. This is very dangerous and my resident care director (RCD) must attempt to resolve this hazardous issue.

Laughter through tears

Caring for my parents at home included managing their medications. I used an automatic 14-day pill dispenser that was round in shape. We jokingly named it the flying saucer. The dispenser was designed to electronically open at programmed intervals, morning and evening. Loading it with the meds was a beast of a job, but it sure simplified the daily distributions. Every two weeks, I took Mom and Dad's pill dispensers, and sat on my bed with two trays and their collection of pill bottles. They both took the common medications for Alzheimer's treatment along with an assortment of other meds and supplements.

All told, I loaded over 200 pills into the two dispensers.

One morning during the busy Christmas season, my dad had taken his pills out of the dispenser (when it opened at the scheduled time) and he placed them on a napkin. That afternoon I realized he hadn't taken them. So I put the pills in a cup and took them into the upstairs kitchen to keep them for reloading the dispenser. The next day, while cooking and talking to my husband about Christmas preparations, I reached down and picked up what I believed to be my daily vitamins.

Half way through taking my vitamins, I looked closely into the bowl only to discover a small blue pill that looked just like my dad's prostate med. My eyes grew as big as that flying saucer! I suddenly knew I had taken several of my dad's meds—including the ones for his dementia. Well, let me just say that I went on a journey I don't ever want to take again!

The pills mishap reminded me that the stress of juggling life when caring for loved ones at home can have a cost. Thankfully, the event caused no harm to anyone. In the end, we had a good giggle in the midst of difficult times.

—Halle

Medication errors are a common problem when families are managing Mom's daily meds. Falls, confusion and agitation can all be caused by skipped meds or meds taken at the wrong time.

A few of the following medication scenarios can be detrimental to Mom's well-being and health.

Drug-drug interactions – The issue of drug-drug interaction may increase or decrease the effects of one or both drugs. This can cause serious consequences. During the winter, Mom may self-treat her flu or cold by using different over-the-counter meds that contain the same compounds as her prescribed medications. Symptoms may worsen or toxicity may develop as a result. Drug-drug interactions can be reduced by periodically updating your mom's records and including her self-care meds as well. Have these records with you when you take Mom to her doctor.

Over use - If Mom needs one tablet a day then two must be better, right? Obviously, this is dangerous thinking.

Improper dose – The bottle may only offer an abbreviation of the dosage and the caregiver may become confused and offer the wrong dosage. For example, the dosage may call for half (SS), but a whole tablet is given, or two eye drops are given rather than the one prescribed eye drop.

Tablet Splitting – Families try to save on the cost of expensive medications by splitting them. Pills formulated to give Mom medication slowly throughout the day may lose this capability if split in half. Also, sometimes families will split every pill in the entire bottle. The problem with this practice is that air degrades the exposed medication and the potency may not be maintained.

3) Home Safety

Falls, toxins and a hazardous surroundings are all part of safety issues you must be concerned about with home care. Communicate with other family members and friends that are familiar with your mom's behavior and routine. Write down everything you can think of that could be a potential hazard.

Does Mom wander or get up at night?

Has she fallen before?

Does she look for food at night?

Does she exit seek and check every door?

Investigate each room (including the bathrooms) for potential hazards and make a note of changes you'd like to make. Adjusting the environment will be more effective than trying to adjust Mom's behavior. Telling Mom to not touch a hot stove is not good enough; you must also adjust the environment. Restrict access to items such as cleaning products, tools, alcohol, forks, knives, scissors, and lighters. Remember that anything can be mistaken as a refreshing drink or a delicious treat.

Disconnect the garbage disposal, install latches on cabinets and drawers and install a video monitoring system and place it in her bedroom, bathroom, kitchen and all exits. Remove bathroom door locks, and install grab bars in the bathroom and shower. Adjust the hot water heater thermostat to below 120F. Keep in mind that Mom may become frustrated because she can't get a cabinet or drawer open. There are many options to make cabinets safe. I have had success exploring cabinet and appliance lock options with the wonderful people at Best Buy and Home Depot.

4) Caregiver Burnout

Studies on families caring for elders in the residence, like the Poulshock and Deimling study, have shown that a large percentage of in-home caregivers (for a loved one with dementia) suffer from stress, illness and clinical depression. Keep in mind; this is typically a 24-hour job, seven days a week. Also, most caregivers do not seek counseling for their depression. The reasons I hear most from in-home caregivers are: "There is no time for counseling", and "As soon as I get some sleep I will be fine." Caregiver burnout is mental, emotional and physical exhaustion. Caregivers often focus so closely on the needs of the one receiving care that they neglect their own health and wellness. As this lack of self-care continues, caregiver's exhaustion often intensifies, impacting different aspects of one's personal lives as well as their effectiveness and compassion that can be offered as a caregiver.

In my initial meeting with the family, I often see family caregivers at their breaking point. I try to be compassionate and empathize with family caregivers. One of the many symptoms of caregiver burnout is irritability. You can actually be mad and not know why you are upset. I try to explain in my initial meeting that many family caregivers are angry for being angry. It is actually possible to be very angry at Mom and yet be angry at yourself for being angry with Mom. (Note: Some readers will be confused by that last statement, but unfortunately, many of you will understand all too well what it means.)

Symptoms of Caregiver Burnout are in some ways very similar to the symptoms of Post-Traumatic Stress Disorder (PTSD).

Symptoms of Caregiver Burnout	Symptoms of PTSD
Withdrawal from friends, family and other loved ones.	Feelings of detachment or estrangement from others.
Loss of interest in activities previously enjoyed	Diminished interest or participation in activities
Changes in sleep patterns	Difficulty falling asleep or staying asleep or restless sleep
Feelings of wanting to hurt yourself or the person for whom you are caring	Reckless or self-destructive behavior
Emotional and physical exhaustion	Hyper vigilance – a state of increased anxiety that causes exhaustion.
Irritability	Irritable or aggressive behavior
Source - Cleveland Clinic https://my.clevelandclinic.org/health/diseases/9225-caregiving-recognizing-burnout	**Source - ADAA** https://adaa.org/understanding-anxiety/posttraumatic-stress-disorder-ptsd/symptoms

Drug and alcohol abuse can also be a common symptom in both examples.

5) Hygiene Issues

Dementia can cause improper hygiene. Mom may forget to shower or may recall that she has just taken a shower, even if it was a memory from many days ago. Fear, trust and depression can be the reasons for not bathing regularly. Mom may fear getting naked in front of a stranger or she may fear for her safety and be afraid of falling. Mom may not trust the person giving the bathing or may not understand the directions being given. It is much easier to say **NO** to something you don't understand than to go along willingly. A few tips to homecare bathing are keeping the bathroom a nice and toasty temperature, play some soft music to relax Mom and do everything very slowly. Talking to Mom in a soothing understanding voice will help to keep Mom calm. Keep moving forward while explaining each step of the process. Cheer Mom on and tell her that she is doing great and how proud you are of her.

Mom may still not cooperate. If you have tried everything including begging, offering rewards and downright blackmail, there's one more method worth trying.. Take Mom's shoes and socks off and start with a foot massage, then gradually work your way to her ankles and calves. Look Mom in the eyes and slowly tell her you will now massage her shoulders. Then take Mom's shirt and bra off, start on her shoulders and back. After a short period of time, again look Mom in the eyes and tell her, "Now that you're half naked we are going to get you washed up, we are going to walk over here and get clean now." Never ask a question where Mom can say no. Always use a confident reassuring tone.

A walk-in shower with a shower chair and shower wand is recommended to have installed. Add a few sturdy hand rails for safety also.

Bad hygiene can cause some serious health problems. Proper hygiene is vital to preventing urinary tract infections (UTI). Seniors can contract a bad UTI because of poor hygiene and dehydration. I visit many potential residents that had to be admitted to the hospital from their home because of a UTI.

8

What is Day Care?

D ay care facilities usually operate during normal business hours five days a week. Some locations offer additional services during evenings and weekends. In general, there are three main types of adult day care centers:

1) Activity based where social interaction is the main focus.

2) Medical care with activities.

3) Dementia care, mental illnesses and developmental disabilities.

There are rare day care facilities that serve all three.

Many of these facilities are affiliated with other organizations, including home care agencies, churches, skilled nursing facilities, hospitals, medical centers, or other senior service providers. The average adult in day care is a 76-year-old female who lives with a spouse or adult children. About 30 percent of these adults have some form of neurological impairment and more than 70 percent require assistance with daily living activities. Regulation of day care facilities is at the discretion of each state, although the National Adult Day Services Association (NADSA) offers several overall guidelines in its standards and guidelines for adult day care. The staff usually consists of a social worker or manager, an activity director and a few certified nursing aides (CNA). Many adult day care centers also rely on volunteers to run various activities. Full kitchens are rare and most meals are catered in for breakfast and lunch.

Three benefits of adult day care:

1) Day care programs can encourage Mom to spend time with others and enhance her self-esteem. Even if Mom has advanced dementia, she should be able to enjoy music and some activities. Adult day care may also delay Mom from moving to an assisted living or memory care.

2) Day care can give you and others who care for Mom a much needed break, possibly enabling you to spend time with your immediate family. You may use a day care so you can go to work, take care of some personal shopping or just relax.

3) Day care is more cost effective than home care in most scenarios. The cost of day care varies significantly between facilities across the country, but still tends to be less than an experienced dementia caregiver. There are additional costs for various services provided which can be included if you ask for an all inclusive arrangement. You can also ask for an estimate after explaining Mom's needs. Keep in mind that day care facilities have a variety of payment structures. Some charge by the hour while others charge by the half or full day.

9

What is Memory Care?

Memory care facilities specifically cater to residents with neurological disorders. Most communities offer private apartments and shared apartments. Location, size and privacy typically drive how the apartments are priced. Supervised care is provided 24 hours a day by staff trained to care for the specific needs and demands of dementia residents. Memory care facilities should offer specialized services that are not available in assisted living facilities. The activity program must be planned to help stimulate the memory of those with dementia. Caregiver training must also include redirection techniques.

There are 2 common types of Memory Care Facilities:

1) Memory Care Unit within an Assisted Living Community (Multi- Level Care)
2) Memory Care Community Only (Stand Alone Memory Care Building)

Memory Care Unit

Also called special care unit (SCU) or secured neighborhood

Many communities offer secure units that are kept locked 24/7. These units are generally smaller in nature and can only be accessed by staff, and visitors who have authorization or a punch code. They tend to be all-encompassing, with living areas, activities, and dining all within the secured location.

Most communities also offer secured courtyards or outside areas in order to give residents the opportunity to spend time in fresh air, while maintaining their safety. A Memory Care Unit generally provides greater supervision and security than the rest of the facility. Memory care needs to be secured because of the threat of elopement. An elopement is when the resident exits the facility and wanders off the property unsupervised. Exit-seeking behavior is one of the biggest threats to a resident with dementia. If the community is doing a great job, your mom will not necessarily look like someone who has dementia. She may easily pass for a visitor.

OPENING THE DOOR FOR THE LADIES

With the help of video surveillance, I have watched a visiting family member, quite innocently; hold the door for a well-dressed woman to exit. As this man has probably done many times before, he held the door for a lady that was exiting a building. The man and the woman smiled at each other, the woman said "thank you" as the man walked in, unknowingly holding the door, allowing a resident to leave the property. How many of us would have the courage to ask a lady that is standing near the exit of a senior facility: "Before I hold the door for you, do you live here?"

—Keith

Stand-Alone Memory Care

Because of the increase in the number of dementia cases and the increased need for quality dementia care, many stand-alone memory care communities have been built in recent years. These communities care only for those with dementia and neurological disorders.

There is great advantage in designing an entire facility to care for those with dementia. All caregivers in the community will be specifically trained for memory care and will have opportunity to become familiar with each resident. Additionally, the memory care facility building design can allow residents to move about safely, always in view of caregivers. Such an arrangement provides for a genuine community of care for each and every resident.

Many communities have a care level system that scales up the cost as increased care is needed. Some communities will advertise low rent rates, but have multiple care rates that are very high. Other communities will have higher rent rates, but only have a few care levels that are less. The average cost of memory care varies from state to state. Costs may include rent, care, a one-time community fee, and monthly ancillary charges that include incontinence products, gloves, hairdresser services, and transportation. A care assessment will be completed to develop a care plan. Most recently, a trend to offer an all-inclusive package has become more prevalent. This program may help some families manage Mom's budget better because the cost of her care will not change for possibly her entire stay.

Here in Atlanta, our competitive analysis confirms that very few communities charge the same way. The monthly cost in this area ranges from $2,300 for a shared apartment to $8,000 for an all-inclusive private apartment. The average monthly cost for rent and care in a memory care facility in Atlanta is approximately $4,400. Medicare does not cover the cost of memory care and Medicaid coverage is limited. There may be some state programs or even federal programs, such as the Veteran's Aid and Attendance benefits that can help cover the cost.

For more information on the VA benefit visit www.veteranaid.org

First impressions

I have learned that in order to be successful you must know your competition. So once a month I tour a competitor's community. We call it "peeking over the fence." Sometimes I schedule an appointment and other times I just walk in. After completing the tour, I have left communities encouraged and happy, while other times I have left discouraged and heartbroken. When entering a memory care community, the welcome I receive from the staff ranges from warm and friendly to open hostility. I look for smiling faces and clean residents. If I am greeted by a caregiver in a friendly way with a smile, that really means a great deal to me. I love to hear a caregiver say, "Is someone helping you?" If you think about it, the caregiver is exhibiting characteristics that you are looking for in a community. You want the community's caregivers to be observant, helpful, polite, courteous, and gracious.

If I walk into a community where I stand around and wait or have to look to find someone, this may tell me that this community is understaffed or possibly just not interested in helping. If I start to walk down a hallway with caregivers refusing to look up or smile, I know this isn't somewhere I would want my parent to live.

—Keith

Giving up the Car Keys

When my mom and dad first moved to Atlanta to live with us, my dad was still driving his car. His executive skills were still intact and it was important to him to keep his independence. Although he had to learn his way around in a new city, he mainly drove to the grocery store, church and a nearby mall. Due to his diagnosis of mild cognitive impairment, we knew it was important to invest in an extensive clinical driving evaluation. The evaluation, which can be costly, was conducted by a certified specialist at an area PT/OT clinic. Thankfully, he passed the test. However, we continued to monitor his driving for the next few years. One day I received a call from a neighbor who had observed my dad driving erratically in the neighborhood. Right away, we scheduled him for a second driving evaluation. The test showed that his driving abilities were still solid but his reasoning was failing him. He wasn't making safe decisions and confusion was creeping in. Dad's general physician was wonderful to help our family by telling my dad he could no longer drive. This was perhaps the most stressful season in our home. Because my dad's short term memory had deteriorated, every day he woke up and asked for the keys. We finally had to sell his car. Many months passed before he stopped looking for his keys and that car. We were relieved, however, that he was safe. It was so painful to see my dad lose his independence. I am pleased to find that many counties now provide seniors with free transport services such as Dial-a-Ride and Dial-a-Bus.

–Halle

10

How do I choose the best Memory Care Community?

Choosing a memory care facility can be emotionally exhausting. However, taking the extra time to research may make a difference to your mom's quality of life. The first, and most important, issue that you need to think about is the needs of your mom. Any memory care community that you choose needs to be able to address the specific requirements unique to your mom, and provide the highest quality of care with compassion. Sometimes families assume a community is right for their loved one because it has a high price and lavish features, but later realize fancy furniture and beautiful landscaping are not at all good indicators of quality care. Families often find that they need to move their loved one to another community, one that, perhaps, less shiny but more appropriate in terms of care or atmosphere.

A beautiful, modern and upscale facility is just as prone to oversights and errors as a community that is 20 years old. Quality of care is not something you can discern just by looking in the door to gauge the mood and whether or not you like how it smells. When you schedule a tour, go with the mind set of "I hope I like this place." Take your time and really get to know the community. I once was assisting a group touring our community, when they sat down in the activity room and told me to go away. They ended up getting involved and truly enjoyed their visit. They then decided to have lunch with the residents. They told me that they could see their Mom living here, and also believed that she would love it.

Always look into the official backgrounds of the communities you are exploring. The office of your local Long-term Care Ombudsman (which you can locate at www.eldercare.gov may tell you about documented issues or problems that local communities have had in the past so that you don't choose a community with a history of substandard care.

Occasionally, a family will visit us for a tour and tell me they were told to write down a list of the most important questions that come to mind concerning a memory care facility. When I ask families what questions they come up with, the answer is usually the same: "Well .... I got nothing ....I don't know what the most important questions are!" My response to them is: "Why should you?" No one can become an expert in memory care overnight and know what questions to ask.

To help families with this dilemma, I put together a list of the best questions to ask and what you should look for during a tour. Read them over and copy down the few that seem to fit your mom's situation.

You can find this at www.parentaldementia.com

Questions to consider asking:

- Can you convince me that Mom will receive the best care here?
- Are the residents grouped by level of dementia or cognitive abilities?
- Will we be able to decorate Mom's apartment?
- Will Mom be able to navigate her way to the dining room and activities?
- Will you escort Mom to the dining room or activities?
- Is the building secure?
- Is there a courtyard?
- Does the staff take residents outside on a daily basis?
- What is the kitchen's health department score?
- What was the score of the last state survey?
- Will family and friends be able to join Mom for meals?
- Can Mom's special dietary restrictions be met?
- Does the care team receive special training on how to manage dementia?
- How often is the care team re-trained?
- Is there a nurse on duty or on call 24 hours a day?
- What situations or conditions would lead to Mom's discharge?
- What is the resident-staff ratio during the day and at night?
- What is the state required resident-to-staff ratio?
- Who will inform the family of any changes in care for Mom?
- Is there transportation to offsite medical appointments available?
- How long has the current management staff been there?
- Does the community offer religious services that Mom would enjoy attending?
- How often are housekeeping and laundry service provided?
- Do you offer headphones for Mom's hearing issues during activities?
- What emergency plans are in place in case of a fire or other such events?
- Is video surveillance used to monitor staff?
- Can I review medical records belonging to Mom?

What you should look for on a tour:

- Does the staff wear uniforms and name tags?
- Is the community well-designed and maintained?
- Are there cameras in the hallways?
- Do the resident's clothes look clean or do they have food stains on them?
- Do the caregivers appear tired and stressed or are the happy and smiling?
- Are residents left on their own just sitting in common areas or in hallways?
- Is the community generally pleasant, clean, and peaceful?
- Is the Activity Room TV on 24/7?
- Are residents parked in front of the TV watching BET or MTV?
- Do you see many residents in their apartments lying in bed?
- Has the medical cart been sitting in the same place unattended for long time?
- Are the caregivers engaged with the residents?
- When you talk to a caregiver, are they friendly?
- Do I get a warm and friendly feeling?

Apartments

When looking for an apartment for Mom you may have a choice of room sizes, floor plan and sometimes location. You may also have to choose between a single or double occupancy apartments for Mom.

Would Mom like a roommate?

Would a roommate like Mom?

Memory care usually will offer studio apartments, one bedroom apartments, double occupancy apartments and couples apartments.

Keep in mind that there are typically large common areas, TV lounges and activity rooms for Mom to spend most of her day, so most residents do not require a large, private two bedroom apartment. Renting a studio apartment instead of a one-bedroom apartment reduces monthly fees by $400 to $1,000 monthly.

A few features to look for that will help keep Mom safe and comfortable are:

- Are handrails installed in the bathroom and hallways within the community?
- Is there ample lighting?
- Is the Flooring made of non-skid materials?
- Is the available apartment free of odor?
- Is the available apartment kept at a comfortable temperature?
- Is there a walk in shower?

I believe the apartment location in the community can be important. If Mom is a joiner and loves activities, try to find an apartment near the activity room. If Mom enjoys her privacy, she may want her apartment near the back of the community. The community may have a beautiful courtyard, so if Mom loves the feel of the sun or enjoys smelling flowers, try to find an apartment near a door leading to the secured courtyard. If Mom isn't mobile, it may be wise to be closer to the dining room and activity room.

Some companies have decided to a build a "communal washing room" for their residents and remove the shower from the apartment bathrooms. Their explanation is that a communal washing room can be better to assist their residents and offer more space for their safety.

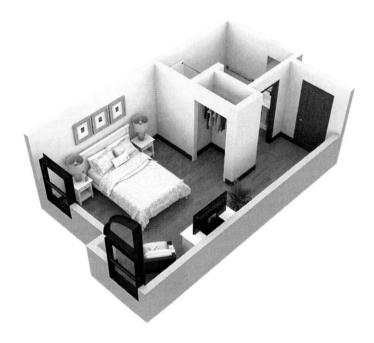

Furnished / Non-Furnished – A furnished apartment can be great if you need to move Mom quickly. If Mom is in the hospital or recovering in a rehabilitation facility, you may want to move Mom directly to the community rather than bringing Mom home and then having to repack and move her belongings to the community. Some memory care communities keep all their available apartments furnished. The idea is to make it as easy as possible for families to move in to their community. All the families have to do is bring pictures, toiletries, clothes and Mom. There are also memory care communities that will loan or rent you furniture until Mom's belongings can be moved to the community.

I have found that the transition into memory care can be different for everyone. In my experience, familiarity helps ease the anxiety that Mom may feel from moving to a foreign environment. An unfamiliar bed and nightstand can actually cause issues with some new residents. Mom may become confused because she thinks she's being asked to sleep in someone else's bed.

Flooring - Memory care apartment flooring typically will be a non carpeted floor. A linoleum or LVT floor is used when safety is a key concern. These types of floors are easy to clean and hygienically appropriate. Also, if Mom uses a wheelchair, she will have a much easier time maneuvering up and down the hallways. With that said, Mom may prefer carpeting.

Bathroom – Look for a large and roomy bathroom. Mom may one day have balance issues and will require help with bathing and transferring to the toilet. The last thing you need is Mom falling because a caregiver could not get in the proper position to assist. The bathroom should also have a sink area that a wheelchair can easily roll up to and position herself somewhat under the counter. If Mom wants to brush her teeth and not have to stand up, the cabinet and counter need to be designed with that in mind.

A walk-in shower should be a requirement. Too many times a resident will not be able to maneuver over even the smallest raised lip entering the shower. This small feature could eliminate a huge fall-risk issue. Imagine placing a 2x4 in front of a doorway and expecting Mom to remember to step over it every time she enters that room.

Finding your Happy Place

Overall, when touring, do you get a sense of happiness or anxiety? Talk to the residents. Watch the residents interact with staff. What do you see? Do the caregivers look like they are enjoying their job? Do you see smiles and laughter or do you see nervousness? In my experience, a well trained care team walks the halls with confidence. They should strike you as experts in caregiving. When a community changes their management team every year, it is frankly not fair to the residents, families or staff. I have interviewed many caregivers that would like to leave their current employer and join my community. When I ask them why they are looking to make a move, they respond, "Too much turnover where I am working." When your supervisor keeps changing, you lose a certain confidence in knowing you're doing what is expected. When expectations change, management styles change, culture changes, attitudes change and when in-house policies change, it leaves the staff bewildered and confused. Confusion causes errors, and errors in a memory care can be dangerous. It is better to choose a memory care that has stability, not only with management, but also with their caregivers.

Caregivers - A memory care community simply cannot be successful without a devoted team of caregivers. In many ways, they are the heart and soul of the community. Caregivers are the difference between a thriving memory care community and a community that always has problems. The caregiving staff in our community is among the best I've ever seen in the industry.

These are the qualities you should look for in all caregivers:

Empathy, Patience, Dependability, Compassion, Reliability, Passion and the Ability to be a Team Player.

Add to these qualities: knowledge, experience, courage and a loving nature and now you have something extraordinary.

Empathy – A great caregiver is someone who is able to cultivate closer bonds by sharing in the happiness or sadness of their residents. When caring for residents, it is essential that a caregiver feel the desire to want to help. By showing empathy, caregivers will let the residents know that they care about them and want to do what they can to help them. This builds trust and eventually calmness in the resident. Empathy helps to put the caregiver in the resident's shoes and see what it might be like to rely on others for help.

Patience – A *good* caregiver will understand that slowing down is a process of aging. A *great* caregiver allows residents to move at their own pace and does not make them feel rushed. When you work with someone who needs care it is important that the caregivers are patient and understanding.

Dependability & Honesty – A great caregiver knows how to work independently. They'll be on time and prepared. Because most care is performed in the residents home or apartment unsupervised, honesty is required. Obviously, theft is never acceptable. Most residents are in a vulnerable position. They trust someone into their home to be near their valuables. A great caregiver is someone who is trustworthy.

Compassion – A *great* caregiver possesses a powerful desire to help seniors. They must be capable of listening to provide companionship. Good communication is the key to all successful relationships and this is especially true when it comes to the relationship a caregiver has with their residents and the resident's families. Being able to compassionately communicate details regarding the resident's care in clear and simple terms builds understanding and trust.

Reliability - A *great* caregiver is someone who can be counted on to be there. If the caregiver commits to their schedule, will the caregiver show up? The entire care team must be reliable and dependable. One of the biggest stressors for a care team is when there are call offs. Working short is when the care team is working their shift with fewer caregivers than reasonably recommended. *This practice is avoided whenever possible because it can be potentially dangerous to the resident's well being.*

Passion - A great caregiver is someone who is passionate about their job and excited about what they do. Their enthusiasm will be evident in how they deal with their assigned residents, who in turn will respond positively to their lively attitude. Passionate caregivers are constantly looking for ways to improve how they perform their jobs, and ultimately, to make the lives of their residents better.

Team Player – I was asked recently to name a pet peeve of mine, I responded, "When I am told that it's not my job or that it's not in my job description." A *great* caregiver is a team player who will do more than their job title states. They put the team's objectives above their own and takes the initiative to get things done without waiting to be asked. They won't passively sit back and see a required care need for the resident and not speak up. Team players take the time to make positive work relationships with other team members a priority and display a genuine passion and commitment toward the entire care team.

Caregiver Ratio - CR refers to how many residents a caregiver is assigned to during a particular shift. If the ratio is 8-1; the caregiver is responsible for eight residents during their shift. A memory care may assign different ratios to each shift. A typical memory care will utilize three shifts per day. The second shift may need a higher level of care than the night shift when almost all the residents are sleeping. For some communities, the numbers will vary only slightly, especially if residents require frequent care at night. However, in most communities, the ratio changes quite dramatically during the nighttime hours. This makes sense because most residents will need significantly less care while sleeping. There are no meals and fewer medications or health needs to monitor as well. At night there may be a few residents who will occasionally need redirection back to their apartments.

If the care ratio is too high and not meeting the residents' needs, the caregivers will look more hurried and stressed out. They won't have time to follow their care plans and offer appropriate care.

During your tour, look at the cleanliness of the residents. Look at their hair, faces, hands, fingernails and clothing. The more residents you notice with messy hair, unwashed or unshaved faces, dirty hands, dirty fingernails, and stained clothing the more concerned you should be with the care ratio that the community has adopted.

Memory Care Key Staff Members include:

Chef / Dining Service Director

"Cooking is the ultimate giving" - Jamie Oliver

Always ask to meet the chef. Mom may have some favorite meals that the chef could cook for her. This little touch could help in Mom's transition. A favorite meal may make your Mom feel special and help the process of moving to a new environment easier. Also, Mom may have food allergies, dietary restrictions or even religious requirements that you could discuss directly with the chef (dining service director). The chef can work to make sure that Mom's nutritional diet is to your satisfaction. Also, check the kitchen's health department score. The State Department of Health Services visits yearly and scores the kitchen's cleanliness and food handling methods.

Activity Director

"It is a happy talent to know how to play" - Ralph Waldo Emerson

The activity director is responsible for leading the community's activity program, which includes the development and implementation of programming geared towards a variety of individual abilities. The AD shows compassion for others and is committed to helping those who needs assistance.

In the morning, I love a loud and busy activity room. The activity room should be moving and grooving to music, exercise, singing or playing games. I recommend staying away from communities that utilize their big screen TV too often. **The TV is not a sitter!** One of the biggest mistakes memory care communities make is to focus on activities that work for the majority of the residents. The Memory Care residents usually will need customized programs. The director needs to know what activities your mom used to enjoy and can still enjoy, and find a way to mix that into the calendar as well. When the activities are not customized, residents will become dissatisfied and feel isolated. Get to know the activity director and share your mom's story. We have our families fill out an extensive biography form that helps the AD understand Mom's history. The AD can then create a more fulfilling activity day for your mom. She will be given opportunities to succeed and this will make her feel good about herself and proud of her new accomplishments.

Maintenance Director

"There is Birth, There is Death, and in between there is Maintenance." – *Tom Robbins*

A good maintenance director will perform routine maintenance and repair work, such as painting, minor carpentry, repair work, changing light bulbs, and various other routine maintenance tasks.

A great maintenance director will perform all the above routine maintenance, but also keep the community free of hazards such as those caused by electrical, plumbing, heating and cooling systems.

I would like to alert you to a trend in the industry that I believe is counterproductive. Facilities are spreading their maintenance personnel over multiple locations and therefore saving payroll dollars. Choose the communities that have full time dedicated maintenance personnel that will be available when Mom needs to have something fixed immediately.

Business Office Manager (BOM)

"Would I rather be feared or loved? The answer is both.
I want people to be afraid of how much they love me'- Michael Scott

The BOM coordinates human resources, payroll, billing and operational processes. As the executive director's right hand, the business office manager is the liaison between families and the executive director. Get to know the BOM as they typically know what is going on in the building better than most employees. They tend to be like the community's bartender or hairdresser; the person with whom the families and employees share all their problems and personal stories. So when you have a question or issue, the BOM could be your go to person.

Housekeepers

"And this mess is so big and so deep and so tall, we cannot pick it up. There is no way at all!" — Dr. Seuss

The housekeepers are important to the overall cleanliness of the community. Ask how many housekeepers they have working daily. A good ratio for a standard memory care community is 20:1. (20 apartments to 1 housekeeper) I am amazed when I am told that there is only one housekeeper and the caregivers have to help clean apartments. This is simply a budget issue and obviously not helping the care of the residents. As a matter of fact, it is probably hurting the care of the residents. It makes no sense that a caregiver cannot spend extra time with a resident who is having a difficult morning because the caregiver has to make sure the room's floor is swept or vacuumed. We teach our caregivers to spend the extra time to get a resident to agree to a bath or to brush their hair. Forcing a caregiver to worry about housekeeping duties is not appropriate, in my opinion.

As for the cleanliness of the community, your first impression can tell you a lot, but you'll also want to do a little detective work. Are corners, baseboards, vents, handrails and windows clean? Check both in the common areas and in the apartments that you visit. You'll also want to find out about the housekeeping arrangements. How often are the rooms straightened up and cleaned? As you are taking your tour, be on the watch for any unusual odors. A bad smell that is confined to a small area may be due to an issue that is easily corrected, but if you notice an unpleasant odor that is throughout the community, it probably indicates a much larger problem.

Resident Care Director (RCD)

"The best way to find yourself is to lose yourself in the service of others."
- Mahatma Ghandi

The resident care director is an integral part of a community's success. The RCD must have the ability to successfully lead team processes and promote a collaborative work environment. Often the Resident Care Director acts as a liaison with hospital personnel, physicians, community organizations, and other health related service agencies to provide care to the residents. They work with their nursing team to coordinate resident care and cultivate an extraordinary group of individuals through hiring, training and scheduling. The RCD and Executive Director set the culture for the community.

You'll want to find out as much as you can about the care offered by the community. Ask about dispensing of medications, bathing options and emergency policies. Ask to review their last survey and their last medication inspection score.

Once you are convinced that your mom will be safe and well cared for, ask them to explain their coordination of care program. Ask how the care plan is communicated to the care team so that assistance for your mom is satisfied appropriately and consistently.

Medical Services - Ask about their policy regarding your family's right to see your mom's medical records and medicine chart. In almost all legal examples, they are not authorized to keep private records on your mom. You have full rights, for example, to see when and which medicines were given to your mom. Care should be the most important element of any community that you are considering for Mom. You'll want to find out as much as you can in this area of care. Ask about things such as dispensing of medications, bathing options, emergency policies and so on. Pay attention to the appearance of residents you encounter on your tour. Are they clean, well-groomed, and appropriately dressed?

Ask about their last survey and their last medication inspection score. Try to schedule a meeting with the resident care director and the executive director. Have a long talk with them. Ask them what they would do in certain scenarios that may occur with your mom. If they can't find the time to meet with you this is a red flag. If you do meet with them, go with your gut. Do they seem knowledgeable, experienced and caring? Ask yourself: Will they take the best care of my mom?

Assessment Plan – The assessment care plan provides direction for individualized care. The care plan is a means of communicating and organizing the actions of the care staff. A memory care community must develop the resident's individual written care plan within 7 to 14 days of admission and require staff to use the care plan as a guide for the delivery of care and services to the resident.

A quality care plan should include a description of the resident's care and social needs. Additionally, the assessment should include Mom's particular preferences regarding care, activities and interests.

The memory care community must show the state evidence of the care plan being updated at least annually and more frequently when Mom's needs have changed substantially. Keep in mind that in most care communities, when additional care is needed so are the care charges.

Remember to ask about each community's policy on care charge increases and what percentages to expect. These charges may need to be factored into your budget.

Ask to be involved in the assessment process. The more you know about the care program, the more you will understand to what extent Mom's disease is progressing.

Coordination of Care – A major issue for some memory care communities is that they are quick to accept new residents only to later discover that they cannot deliver proper care to them. Successful care of your Mom will depend on how well the resident care coordinator communicates assignments to her care team. The resident care director and the executive director should also discuss your mom's needs before accepting her as a new resident. Finally, you will want to ask the resident care director and executive director one direct question: Can this community take care of my mom?

Nurse Practitioner – Because it is difficult to find a doctor to make a house call, many memory care communities utilize a nurse practitioner.

The nurse practitioner will diagnose and treat residents. Their responsibilities may include: managing high blood pressure, diabetes, depression and other chronic health problems, performing comprehensive and focused physical examinations, diagnosing common acute illnesses and injuries, ordering and interpreting diagnostic tests such as X-rays and EKGs and other laboratory tests, as well as prescribing medications and therapies.

Utilizing a nurse practitioner that specializes in dementia care and dementia medication can be a great addition to Mom's care. If Mom needs a physicians order for a new medication or an X-ray the NP can order it the same day. Also, a nurse practitioner can save you time from running to doctor appointments because the NP can visit your Mom right where she lives.

Along with the nurse practitioner, there are additional health care professionals that are not employed by the memory care community who may interact with your mom. The community will contract additional care professionals to visit monthly or quarterly. These care professionals that will make house calls include; dentists, podiatrists, neurologists, X-ray technicians and even mental health therapists.

Survey Score - One of the items that is often an afterthought when considering assisted living and long-term care is how many, if any, violations and/or citations has the facility received during a particular period of time? This consideration could perhaps be one of the most enlightening discoveries you make, and might help you to further narrow down your choices, and highlight others. Most states require that senior care facilities, such as assisted living and memory care communities, be inspected annually, semiannually, or at specified times between one and two years. State licensing and survey teams are usually made up of nurses, social workers, sanitarians and public health officials. The number of surveyors per team is between one and five. Facility surveys include both direct observation of and interviews with residents, staff, and family members. In addition, a thorough review is given to resident, staff, and facility records. Survey teams confirm that a resident assessment has been performed properly and that care plans have been developed. They also check facility records as well as verify appropriate licensure documentation.

Most assisted living and memory care communities have been cited from time to time.

A good community will resolve minor issues quickly. Keep an eye out for neglectful communities that are cited for major infractions and fail to fix their issues quickly.

Medication Management Score - Does the community audit their medication department? Medication management is a complex process of reconciling, monitoring, and assessing the medications that Mom is prescribed. A community must assure compliance with a specific medication schedule while also ensuring the individual avoids potentially dangerous drug interactions and other complications.

Medication errors are one of the reasons that families choose to move their loved one from their home to a memory care community. Unfortunately, assisted living facilities and memory care communities are also known to make medication errors.

Medication errors are defined by the National Coordinating Council for Medication Error Reporting and Prevention as being any preventable event that may cause or lead to inappropriate medication use or patient harm while the medication is in the control of the health care professional, patient, or consumer. Medication errors resulting in harm to elderly patients can be caused by negligence, failure to follow directions, malice on the part of caregivers or relatives, improper labeling, and many other factors. Approximately

1.3 million people in the United States are harmed each year from incidents stemming from medication errors.[14]

There are two major concerns when it comes to administering medicine in a Memory Care Community.

1) **Accuracy** - Staff must accurately administer medications. This means giving the right medicine at the right time to the right resident and documenting it appropriately.

2) **Proper Medication** - The prescribing doctors must prescribe the best medications for each resident with regards to all interactions and allergies.

Therefore, many memory care communities have an oversight program to audit the medication procedures and policies. Over 70 percent of communities have a pharmacy or physician that reviews the medications that residents receive for appropriateness.

The oversight body then provides a score for how the community is operating their medication program. The oversight body will also test and observe the certified medication technicians and LPNs to help validate that their training has been useful and successful. Education and communication are the keys to medication management in memory care communities. Most residents take several medications and visit more than one prescribing doctor.

Coordinating multiple pharmacies, managing over the counter drugs vs. prescribed medications vs. supplements and dealing with multiple doctors tend to make medication management a challenge. Memory care communities that utilize an oversight program will catch all or most conflicting medications that could cause severe harm to the residents. An oversight body like a pharmacy or a doctor will help reduce medication errors. If the community is not familiar with this practice they may be setting themselves up for a tremendous fall. You may want to stay away from communities that refuse to audit their medication department.

---

5 Signs of a Great Medication Program

1) Medications are dispensed at the appropriate dosage and time.

2) Medications are well documented.

3) Medications are cross-referenced for specific allergies and adverse drug reactions.

4) If a drug reaction occurs, prompt attention is given and correction plans are immediately enacted to prevent harm to the resident.

5) The medication management program is routinely reviewed and if needed, improved in a timely manner.

24-hour phone – May I reach a supervisor from the community at anytime of the day or night? If I want to call and talk to Mom, do I need for her to have a phone or may I call the community? Typically, the community should have a method for you to be able to talk to your mom.

Pharmacy - When the community takes over your mom's medication management, they will be responsible to make sure that Mom is receiving the right meds at the right time and in the right quantity. The community will also take on the responsibility of ordering, keeping inventory and safely storing Mom's medications. Typically a community works with a pharmacy where they can order medications and have them delivered to the community in a timely manner. Mom's medications will be delivered to the medication technician in a bubble pack card that is identified as her medications. Make sure your community is using a pharmacy that will work with your insurance. Also, be prepared to pay slightly more for Mom's medications due to the pharmacy preparing your mom's medications in the bubble pack card.

The Value of a Pharmacist

In our family's experience, we have found that many doctors are quick to prescribe a go to medication that they like. However, that medication may or may not be the best choice for your mom. When it comes to prescription meds, we have found our pharmacist to be the one to dispense a wealth of knowledge and insight on how medications work together, the potential side effects of certain meds, and "generic" meds that do the same as the name brand. This can save you hundreds of dollars. We love our pharmacist and will even call him from home to ask questions. Take the time to find a friendly, knowledgeable pharmacist who will take the time to talk with you. You'll be glad you did!

–Halle

Rent and Fees

Calculating Mom's long-term care expenses can often be tricky due to the unforeseeable care needs that occur with the advancement of dementia. This typically leads to more costs. The first cost to consider is the monthly rent of the particular apartment that you have chosen for your mom. When selecting a community be aware of additional fees that could be tagged on to the monthly rent. Many fees are adjustable and negotiable. Here is a list and explanation of the fees that you might see on your bill:

Care charges – Will the community's rates be affordable for the foreseeable future?

Typically, care charges are added as Mom's dementia progresses. So it is important to select a community that Mom can live in as long as possible without cost becoming an issue and thus forcing her to move.

Most communities will offer a tiered system to charge for care costs. The community will charge you more as Mom's care increases. Every 60– 90 days the resident care director will complete a new assessment that will assess your mom's care needs.

The RCD will then meet with the executive director and discuss all of the activities of daily living (ADLs) that are required for your mom. If your mom's care increases, a decision may be made to increase her care charges. These increases could be a few hundred dollars more a month. In some communities there are only two to three care levels and in others you may discover eight to 12 care levels. Unfortunately, this means the cost increases would stretch out for many months or years. There are a few communities that will offer an all-inclusive program. This program offers a rate that will take the cost of care and include it in the rent for an agreed upon length of time. This program can offer the most cost-effective plan in the long run, but not always. I recommend that before you sign papers for move in, ask for both options.

Examples of these options might include:

Rent + Level 2 Care = $3,900.00 + $500.00 = $4,400.00 a month

All-Inclusive Care = $4,600.00 a month

Incontinence - Ask if the community has an additional incontinence charge. Many communities include incontinence in their care charges while others claim to be à la carte. If Mom becomes incontinent, several communities will charge for the additional housekeeping and bathing that will be necessary to keep Mom's living situation dignified.

Bathing – Bathing is typically included in the care charges. The ADL assessment is either independent or assistance needed. Watch out for communities that have figured out a way to add an additional charge for bathing assistance. If Mom is an independent bather, it makes sense that there should not be a charge for bathing. What if there is no shower in Mom's apartment and now she needs to be escorted to the bathing area and supervised for her safety? Also, make sure you are aware of how many showers Mom is scheduled to have every week. If Mom has incontinence issues, try to negotiate a rate that includes showers as needed.

Hair Salon – The community's hair salon will typically adjust their prices to fit the needs of their residents. Expect a weekly charge of approximately $20 - $50 added to your bill from the hairdresser. If needed, you can adjust the frequency of visits.

Transportation – Many communities include scheduled transportation in their monthly rent while others charge for all transportation. Ask up front for an explanation of their transportation policy and schedule.

Dining Service – Typically three meals and two or three snacks are included in the rent. What is not always included is if Mom prefers to eat in her apartment. The community may charge you a tray service to serve your Mom in her apartment. Make sure you have a discussion about this before you get a surprise. Also, check to see if the community charges for guest meals.

DINNER WITH TIM'S NEW GRANDMOTHER

I once had to forgive a $200 guest meal charge from a resident's bill. One of my residents invited a young man named Tim who was attending a nearby college to have dinner with her and her friends. Tim had been hired to entertain the residents with his singing and guitar playing. The resident quite innocently introduced him as her grandson Timmy, as he bore the same name. Not wanting to embarrass her, Tim went along and stayed to have dinner with his "new grandmother." Tim so enjoyed the visits that he dined with her and her table mates after each performance. When the resident's family received the monthly bill, they asked about the mysterious guest meal charge. I explained that their son Timmy eats dinner with their mom on occasion. They responded, "What are you talking about? Timmy is in the Army overseas!"

So of course, I waived the guest meals and waited to speak to "Timmy."

After a lengthy chat with Tim, I discovered that he treasured the dinner conversation with his adopted grandmother so much that he came weekly to visit her. The happy ending to the story is that her family welcomed Tim's kindness and he went on to become a regular volunteer at our community. In fact, Tim volunteered for the next three years and even switched his major to nursing. He now works as a regional director of nursing in assisted living. And, no, we never charged him for any guest meals.

–Keith

Utilities – Ask if all utilities are included. Cable, Wi-Fi and phone are typically not included.

Ambulance – If Mom needs to go to the emergency room for any reason, the transportation to the hospital is not usually included in the community's rent.

Ambulance services can range from free to extremely expensive. If you are in a city where services are covered by taxes then there is no cost to Mom. For residents without health insurance your cost will range from $300 to $1,500, plus mileage. The ambulance cost can depend on whether the trip is for an emergency or a scheduled transport, how many miles the resident travels and whether basic life support or advanced life support was needed.

Rent Increases – Room and board rates are still subject to annual rate increases. On occasion, communities will ask for rent increases. You can expect approximately a 2 percent to 8 percent yearly rent increase throughout Mom's stay. Yearly increases in salaries, fuel, and utilities have an adverse effect on the community's working budget. Try to negotiate an increase cap amount before you complete Mom's move-in paperwork.

Care Supplies – Not all care supplies will be included in your mom's care package. There may be an additional charge for gloves, Depends, wipes, bed pads, and pull ups. If you are able to buy your own supplies, the cost for the supplies will typically be less. Keep in mind that your time is also valuable and you may have to drive a few places to get your supplies. To save money, I suggest ordering all your supplies on line in large quantities, storing them at home and delivering to Mom when needed. For a few more dollars, try negotiating with the community a fixed monthly cost for all needed supplies and let them be responsible for everything. It will be worth it in the long run.

Amenities

Memory care communities may offer amenities such as walking paths, beauty/barber shops and courtyards. Decide which amenities are especially important to you, and ask to see them on your tour. Check for handrails in hallways and bathrooms. Are the floors made of non-skid material and is the carpeting firm enough for ease of walking? Are cupboards easy to reach? Are there sprinklers and smoke detectors? Are common areas, hallways and rooms accessible to wheelchairs and walkers? If the community has more than one floor, are there elevators to the upper levels? How do residents in wheelchairs exit the community in case of an emergency?

Once the major questions have been answered, remember to trust your instincts. Do you feel comfortable and at ease? Is this somewhere that you could really see your mom thriving? If the answer to these questions is yes, then follow your heart. Choose a community where you can see your mom happy, respected, loved and comfortable.

The following are a few amenities that I believe are important and should be highlighted.

Meals - Make sure you check out the dining options. Visit the dining room and stay for a meal if possible. You'll want to find out about the serving schedule and procedures. How many meals are provided each day? Is Mom allowed to dine in her room? What arrangements are there for family and friends who may visit? If your mom has any dietary restrictions, it's important to find out if they can accommodate. Can the community serve mechanical soft or puree meals if needed? Are caregivers trained in feeding? Is the community licensed to feed their residents? What is the kitchen's latest health score? Just like a restaurant, the state health department will score the community's kitchen.

Secured Environment – Safety is extremely important. A high level of safety will contribute positively towards Mom's transition. Every memory care community needs to be secured from a resident wandering away off the community's property. Make sure that the community has a plan in place to protect Mom from eloping from the building.

Many communities also have policies to keep residents' apartment doors closed and locked. The public reasoning is to insure your mom's privacy and security. While security may be part of the reason, another significant reason for this policy is to prevent wandering residents walking in and making themselves at home in the wrong apartment. Also, residents with dementia will often hunt and gather all types of items. One day I was alerted that 12 residents were missing their glasses. We found them in a very sweet resident's apartment. She had decided to keep them safe for all her friends in her cabinet.

Keeping the door closed is also a way to keep the smell of a resident's incontinence from reaching the hallway. I believe that the risk of a resident falling and not being seen because of a closed door is greater than dealing with wandering residents and some temporarily lost belongings. Also, if the care team and housekeepers are trained properly on incontinence product disposal along with the appropriate resident bathroom assessments, closed doors are not necessary.

Activity Schedule – The monthly activity schedule should be posted for you to review during your tour. Go through each day and look for the activities that Mom would enjoy. Ask to have the activity schedule emailed to you if you decide to have Mom move in. Look closely at the weekend activities. Check to see if the community will have significant activities scheduled on the weekends. Ask if these activities are done consistently. Some communities will rely on volunteers to lead activities on Saturdays and Sundays.

Pet Therapy - Studies have suggested that pets are good for us, even offering health benefits such as lowering our blood pressure and heart rate, reducing the stress hormone, cortisol, and boosting levels of the feel-good hormone, serotonin and oxytocin. Having our four-legged friends in a memory care community is a perfect fit. Pets bring great benefits to all of us, including companionship, unconditional love, and responsibility. By nature, pets are not critical and they are not judgmental and for residents with dementia, those qualities make them a fantastic companion.

Music Therapy – I can't imagine that anyone who works in memory care doesn't love music therapy. Music therapy gives Mom an opportunity to interact socially and can actually change her mood from sad to joyful. I have found that music through wireless headphones help my residents become more social and seem more engaged and focused. The trick is to play the music that Mom loves and is familiar to her. Music therapists that work with dementia residents describe seeing people who appear to wake up when the sounds of familiar music fills their ears. Often, after months or even years of not speaking at all, residents will begin to talk and even sing again. We have also found that music therapy can help us redirect residents who have exit seeking tendencies. In addition, we found that the lyrics to gospel music seem to awaken their memories of those familiar and favorite melodies. I once put a Catholic Mass on TV and gave the wireless headphones to many of the residents and turned up the volume. Frankly, I could only stand there with my mouth open. Many of the residents who rarely communicate began to respond back to the priest singing "Peace be with you." There were about seven residents who were singing out in response, "And also with you."

Sweet Music to the Soul

Music had a special place in my dad's life. His mom played the piano when he was young and in college he joined a barber shop quartet. For many years, he loved joining his quartet buddies, dressing up in his red skimmer and vest, and singing four-part harmony. Then there were the hymns that our family sang every week at church. My mom and dad didn't know it at the time, but they were building a reservoir of music memory deep inside their hearts and minds. When my family would visit their memory care community for Sunday morning sing-along, we were often amazed how the residents knew the lyrics by heart. As my mom and dad began to decline and, sadly, began to lose their words, we were happily surprised to see that they could still sing the words to the hymns that were rooted down inside them. And, when the oldies were played, my dad belted out every barbershop tune like it was still 1950.

Perhaps the most amazing moment arrived toward the end of my mom's life. When she became restless and agitated in the weeks before her passing, she found extraordinary comfort in the hymns we downloaded onto an iPod and played in her apartment throughout the day. She would immediately enter into a place of rest and peace as the music washed over her. I surely hope this generation will fill their hearts and minds with beautiful music that will bring sweetness to their souls in their winter years to come.

—Halle

Video Surveillance – Safety for residents is the prime reason for wanting video surveillance in the memory care community you choose.

The reasons for these safety concerns include:

1) **Caregiver competency** – Surveillance can be used in training as teaching points.

2) **Neglect of residents** – Surveillance can help discover a resident left alone in a locked wheelchair unable to move.

3) **Safety in the event of an accident or to prevent an accident** – Cameras can help prevent wandering residents from entering unsupervised areas as well as investigating how to help prevent a resident from falling.

4) **Internal investigations** – Cameras can uncover if any employee is engaging in any form of dishonesty in the community. Theft is a problem in many residential care facilities, and memory care is no exception. Unfortunately, it is not unheard of for residents to have their possessions stolen. Having a camera in place can offer a deterrent to theft. When a family member or caregiver brings to my attention that something is missing from a resident's apartment, we first think that a staff member did it. Over the years I have found that the staff is only about 20 percent to blame. I have worked long enough to have seen almost everything when it comes to missing resident belongings. I now look at staff, other residents, family members, equipment delivery personnel and medical people. I have found that sometimes wheelchairs seem to disappear when a certain rehabilitation equipment company is in the community. They may come to pick up a bed and a wheelchair, but on the camera I watch them try to leave with a bed and two chairs. Of course, I am sure that it was only by mistake. On another occasion, the surveillance found a visiting doctor walking out of an apartment holding a resident's diamond bracelet.

Communities that Use Security Cameras

Handing your Mom over to the care of a memory care community can create feelings of uncertainty and perhaps even distrust. After all, there are stories of residents who may become confused and mistakenly walk into the wrong apartment and pick up another person's belongings. In fact, personal belongings can be moved around from time to time. Typically, there is a logical story behind the missing items. Memory care communities with video surveillance are locations that are going the extra mile to provide a safe environment for everyone. Senior communities are not required to provide this type of security but the ones that do can keep a sharp eye on 24-hour activity and provide superior security, which establishes a base level of calm and peace for everyone in the community.

Employee safety - Exits and entrances that are monitored by cameras will help protect staff and residents from possible intruders. A typical med room will have medicine and narcotics that may be worth a significant amount of money on the street.

THINGS DO GO MISSING

I remember the first time that a family member came to my office to tell me that her Mom's property was missing. A daughter of a resident was upset with me because her Mom's Nintendo video game console was "stolen." The daughter was so upset that she yelled at me for a solid 10 minutes. I let her get her frustration out and I then asked her. "When did you notice it missing?" She replied, "Well, it was here yesterday!" I told her to give me a minute while I pulled up the video of that hallway. The camera only records when there is movement so pinpointing who removed the console from the apartment would not take very long.

About five minutes later, I asked the woman to come over and view the computer screen. I asked her to tell me who this young man that was walking out of her Mom's apartment holding a grey box with cords hanging from it. The daughter looked at the screen and laughed, "Oh geez .... That's my son; he must have borrowed it and forgot to tell me."

–Keith

Handrails - Handrails in hallways are code driven in skilled nursing homes, but the codes are more lenient in assisted living, memory care, and independent living environments. Often, a lean rail or palm rails are best for an arthritic hand, while a standard round handrail may be more difficult to grasp because of its narrow and unfamiliar shape. The handrails that Mom can lean on with arthritic hands seem to be the safest and most successful of all types of handrails.

Typical round handrails can actually contribute to and possibly cause a fall if Mom's hands cannot grasp the railing while walking.

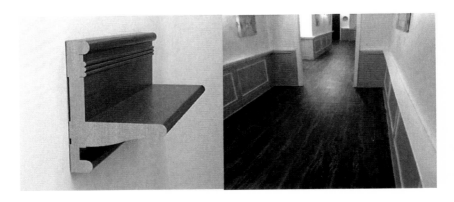

Family Nights – Ask if the community has events that bring families together. Not all communities can offer family nights because of budget or resident acuity. It can be psychologically beneficial for families to talk to others that have similar issues. Sitting with another family that has a loved one in the same community to chat with can help. It sometimes can resembles a mini support group.

Holiday Dinners – Picking Mom up from the community and taking her home to have Thanksgiving Dinner with the family seems like a great idea, until it's not. Sitting at the table, Mom may become confused, scared and embarrassed. Having your Thanksgiving meal at the community is a much safer undertaking. Ask if the community offers holiday dinners to their families.

The Community Reputation

A challenge for families who are searching for a memory care community is that it's not always easy to find information about the licensing and background of the communities that they are exploring. At this time, only a few states post their memory care health department scores online. California, for one, inspects every few years and typically doesn't put the results online. Therefore, you should ask the executive director for the community's record of fines and violations. Most memory care communities should have their last State Survey available for your review.

While there is a national nursing home website to view licensing and audit histories of **Medicare** approved nursing homes, there is no such website (that I am aware of) for **private pay** memory care communities. That's because memory care is regulated at the state level, as opposed to nursing homes, which are regulated at both the state and federal level. A Place for Mom provides a list of assisted living state licensing websites across the U.S.

www.aplaceformom.com/blog/checking-assisted-living-violations-07-26-2013/

Also try reaching out to the Alzheimer Association, Hospital Discharge Nurses, Social Workers, Bloggers, Dementia Support Groups, Referral Services, and Web Site Reviews for more information on the community's reputation.

www.medicare.gov/nursinghomecompare/search.html

11

What do I do after Mom moves to a Community?

I am always asked if the family should stay away for a period of time while Mom gets adjusted and transitions into the daily schedule of the community. My response is always the same "You know your mom better than anyone so we will support you in any decision." Some communities have a set policy of asking families to stay away for a few days so Mom can transition quicker. I have looked at the studies and believe that there is really no basis for this policy. With any neurological disorder, there is typically no normal benchmark and therefore there should not be a set policy concerning family interaction. With that said, I believe that in the case of a resident with exit-seeking tendencies, the family should consider the confusion that might come from taking Mom out frequently for meals and birthday parties. This can lead to undue stress for Mom. It can also add stress to the care team as they will need to constantly redirect her away from wanting to leave.

Conversely, if the family decides to stay away and not visit, Mom could feel abandoned and depressed which could cause additional anxiety and frustration. From my experience, the best practice is for the family to visit Mom, show their love for her and agree to have a positive and supportive attitude toward her new apartment.

There are also studies on the best way to spend quality time with Mom. These studies of how to visit Mom tend to contradict themselves. Some recommend the family to visit sporadically, not at a set time or on a set day. Other studies suggest keeping your visits consistent by visiting the same day and time.

Frankly, I believe you should try to visit Mom at a time of day that is good for her, which can lead to a better visit. Mom may really love morning exercises and not want to visit with you at that time. Or, she may enjoy you joining her by exercising next to her or just sitting nearby to cheer her on.

Choose a time when agitation is low. When visiting, don't expect much and try to keep your family's expectations low. Mom might be feeling unsettled, confused or even irritable. She might not even be up for a visit on a given day. Arrive expecting little in terms of any kind of meaningful conversation. Be ready to do most of the talking and build in some quiet time to just sit and be together.

Resist the urge to fill that silence with conversation. Sometimes it is easier to just hold hands and sit quietly. Our caregivers will occasionally gather to watch one of our residents holding hands with her son in our gazebo.

If Mom is agitated during your visit, take a walk and come back, or just cut the visit short and try again another day. Mom's agitation can be attributed to many things such as confusion, a reaction to a medication, or even frustration with an unexpected change in the daily routine.

If Mom falls asleep during your visit, let her sleep. Alert a caregiver that you're leaving so they can watch over Mom.

I have witnessed many families that visit frequently and truly love seeing Mom while other families are filled with torment because Mom may not recognize them immediately or isn't able to meet their expectation of a normal conversation. I see families feeling guilty because Mom may cry or appear sad when they are saying goodbye. Unfortunately, families also feel guilt for their perceived failure to keep Mom at home. A daughter may say, "If I was a better caregiver we could have kept Mom at home." I want to tell them, "You are a great caregiver...you haven't failed." Everyone's situation is different, so it's not fair to compare yourself to others. Moving Mom to a memory care doesn't mean that you've failed to take care of her. It means you're making a smart decision to get her the level of care she needs. It is only hurtful to you and your family to dwell on negative thoughts and feelings about a decision that you were forced to make for Mom's optimum well-being.

Understanding where the guilt is coming from gives you the chance to remind yourself about the reality of the situation. With time, you'll be able to fully accept the decision.

Put Mom's Name on Everything

One day I purchased eight pairs of cotton pants for my mom and placed them in her closet. When I returned to visit my mom and dad, I looked inside the closet and surprisingly found that all her pants were missing! I soon learned that the night shift had washed her clothes and accidentally put her pants away in three different apartments. Because I had failed to mark the pants with her name, I had to go on a long hunt for the missing items. The next time I visited, I came armed with a permanent marker and fabric name tags ready to tackle the job of tagging all my parent's belongings. While typically no one has ill intent, personal items can be misplaced due to the confusion experienced by some of the residents, or in this case, a staff mishap. I would advise that you err on the safe side and keep your most precious and valuable items safe at home and label all your mom's clothing and personal items that might accidentally be relocated to another place in the building.

—Halle

12

What should I expect from the Community after we move in?

By Halle Eskew

As the caregiving daughter to two parents who struggled with dementia for more than a decade, I learned firsthand what to expect from a memory care community. Caring for my parents began back in my home town where my dad was first diagnosed with early stage dementia or mild cognitive impairment. After many months of traveling back and forth between cities, our family decided to move my parents closer to where we lived. At the time, there were few resources or people to give advice on how to find the right place for them to live that would suit their needs in the early stages of dementia. We relied on the few books available on the topic of Alzheimer's and visits to senior care communities (most of which were simply selling their properties).

We initially considered moving my parents to an assisted living with memory care community near our home. Cost was a driving decision that made it easy to eliminate a few of the choices. Thankfully, my mom's long-term care insurance would help out with the costs. Our first instinct was to find a well-appointed community within budget that my mom would enjoy. She always loved art, architecture and gardens.

So, we reasoned, if we found a community that was upscale, then it meant the managers and the caregivers must be great as well. My brother drove from out of state and joined me on our search. We uncovered nearly a dozen communities that were filled with beautiful furniture and smiling caregivers.

We still weren't sure the best way to determine the right choice for my parents. All our searching came to an end after our family decided to move my mom and dad into a home where my family would live and care for them.

After nearly five years of building wonderful memories with Mom and Dad at home, it was time for them to receive care we could no longer give them despite around-the-clock caregivers we had hired. My mom had declined dramatically after an emergency gallbladder surgery and my dad's dementia was advancing as he became increasingly confused and agitated. We renewed our search for a memory care community nearby. While we were still focused on a lovely setting for my mom, the primary concern was to find a place near our home so we could visit them often.

The pathway that led us to the community where my dad lives today was a long and emotional one. He is not living in the first memory care community we found for my parents, but the fourth one! It took four moves until we learned what we needed to know: the best memory care community is often not the fanciest one. There is a standard of caregiving found in the best places. The people in these facilities treat the residents as they would want to be treated. Shortly after we moved my parents into the fourth community, my mom began to receive the personal attention and exceptional care that had eluded us for so long. Sadly, she had already begun to decline at the time we moved Mom and Dad. She was entering her final stage of dementia just before she arrived at this devoted and compassionate community. Within two months, my mom passed away, ending her painfully difficult battle with dementia.

My hope is that your family will not have to move Mom four times before you find the right community for her. Our reasons for moving my parents were largely due to issues that we were disappointed to find in some of the most beautifully-appointed memory care communities.

Insufficient activities

We first moved my parents to a cozy, elegant personal care home complete with gardens and the artistic design I envisioned my mom would enjoy. The residence even provided fresh home cooked meals and large bedrooms for each of its 12 residents. Best of all, it was fairly close to our home. Within 24 hours I knew this was not the right place for my parents. While the surroundings were attractive, my dad was not content with the laid-back atmosphere and lack of planned activities to engage him. He quickly became agitated and disruptive. We moved them out immediately.

Poor Management

The second move was to a more traditional memory care community that was closer to our home. Our first impression was that this community appeared to have it all: updated design, plenty of activities to occupy my parents, and happy and caring employees. Initially, all seemed well. My parents were getting along with other residents and always had something to do. Slowly, during the course of a few months, I discovered that employees were leaving. First, the activity director left. Later, it was the executive director, followed by several CNAs who departed. Within one year, the community experienced almost 100% employee turnover. Families also began to move their parents from the property. I soon became aware that many of the caregivers were unhappy and poorly trained in dealing with dementia residents. It was time to leave again.

Negligence

We were hopeful that the third move was the charm. After yet another search, we placed my parents in a sister property of the former community. This place looked to be under better management, and the employees seemed to have held their positions for a longer time and appeared happy in their jobs. The selling point was when we met the activity director who would be heading up the brand-new wing where my parents would live. Her enthusiasm and genuine desire to care for the residents was remarkable. We soon moved them in and found the activity director to be everything we had anticipated. Every day she engaged the residents in hands on activities that they thoroughly enjoyed. All the residents seemed to be receiving ample love and attention. There was laughter and contentment among the residents. The activity director even texted images of my parents participating in activities so I would feel a part of their daily routine. We were thrilled...until the day we weren't. Our wonderful activity director, like those before her, left her job after one year. Her replacement was, in every way, the opposite of her. The person who replaced her was uncaring, unoriginal and in many ways disconnected emotionally from the residents. Her job was clearly just a pay check for her.

Over the course of the year, the replacement activity director became more and more disenchanted with her job to the point of neglect. The final blow was when my mom became repeatedly diagnosed with a urinary tract infection. On one visit to my parents, Mom was complaining loudly. The activity director looked at me and glibly said, "Her dementia is just progressing. She's not eating much and she just yells a lot." My antenna went up and I knew in my daughter heart that she was being neglected. Upon further investigation, I discovered that she had been on a round of antibiotics for her UTI but the medical technicians had failed to administer the low-dose prophylactic antibiotics that she needed to prevent a relapse infection. The infection had recurred and was being ignored. Furthermore, they attempted to prevent me from seeing and obtaining copies of her medical records, even though I had a legal right to see them and receive copies. I immediately moved my parents to their fourth community. Right away, I had her transported to a hospital to receive intravenous antibiotics. Her pain quickly subsided and within a week she returned to her new community with Dad.

What to expect from a quality community

Within a few weeks, I knew my parents fourth memory care residence was unlike any we had known. Our family began to believe that this community was possibly the gold standard. It wasn't the fancy carpet. The carpet was old and needed replacing (it has since been replaced). It wasn't their facility (it was decades old.) It wasn't the large gathering spaces. There were a couple of mid-size rooms for residents to congregate. It wasn't their spacious bedrooms (they were on the small side). What made this place special are the things you should expect from an assisted living or memory care community after you move your mom in.

Communication starts at the top

In the previous communities, the communication I received was minimal at best and deceptive at worst. I first made an appointment with Keith Galas, the executive director of the memory care community where my mom and dad eventually moved (for what would be their fourth and final location). When I arrived to meet Keith, he greeted me with a huge smile, a warm heart, and an eager desire to hear my story. We met in a small conference room where he gave me well over an hour of his time to hear me talk about my parents and our difficult journey. He shared his vast experience with dementia patients, his knowledge of the industry, the type of training he had acquired, and the extensive training that his caregivers received. I had never met a memory care director with such an enthusiastic outlook and depth of knowledge. It was clear that he knew the senior care and dementia care industries and that he cared deeply about his community. I truly felt that he was listening to me. He addressed all my concerns by explaining to me how their community was different.

From the beginning, I have been kept in the loop on everything going on with my parents (and now my dad)—from issues regarding their medicines, eating, health, and behaviors. I have been on the receiving end of consistent communication from the medical technicians, the caregivers, and the administrative staff. It is amazing how much better your mom is treated if the people giving the care are willing to treat you as a partner in the process. You should expect a quality community to contact you whenever there is a concern with your mom. If there is an emergency you should be contacted immediately, and for non-emergencies, within 24 hours. I remember when a kind medical technician named Toni accidentally dropped my dad's false teeth after she had cleaned them one night. A tooth was chipped when they hit the floor. She contacted me the next morning, practically in tears as she apologized for her mistake. I assured her that it was only an accident and the teeth could easily be repaired. I was touched by her sincere concern and her honest admission of the small accident. I knew this was a relationship of trust. A foundation of trust is what you should expect at Mom's community.

Caring for the caregivers

I soon learned that Keith's caregivers had been with him, in some cases, for many years. It was exciting to hear that the caregivers were treated like family and were respected by the management and beloved by the residents' families. I knew this was a major part of what I wanted to see in a community. In many cases, if caregivers are not supported, appreciated and recognized, they will not be devoted, happy and motivated to do their work. I was pleased to discover, for example, that families were allowed to anonymously donate money to a Christmas fund that would be divided among the caregivers. Many communities will only allow you to write caregivers a thank you card but not provide gifts or monetary donations. Ultimately, unappreciative treatment of caregivers leads to attrition. The job of these caregivers is physically and emotionally taxing, and I have seen that families are eager to show them love and support. You should expect to see a community filled with caregivers who have been employed there at least a year or two, perhaps longer. In the past two and a half years that my dad has been living in this community, I have frequently heard the caregivers and medical technicians comment that the residents are like their "children." This was demonstrated on one occasion by a medical technician that drove through a treacherous snowstorm to make sure she arrived to work on time to care for the residents. Their heartfelt commitment is unmistakable. Some of the caregivers are caring for their own mom or dad who are living at home and continue their jobs when they come home from work. These sacrifices are a hallmark of true care angels, and these remarkable caregivers should be at the top of the list of what you should expect at the community you choose for Mom.

Waiting lists are a good sign

I was surprised to learn that there were as many as 44 residents in Keith's community when it is filled to capacity (which is typical). While this seemed to me like a large number, the community ranks above state standards in caregiver to resident ratios. You should expect the director of a community to thoroughly vet families interviewing for a spot. The director should make sure that the community is a good fit for Mom and that Mom is a good fit for the community. The caregivers at Keith's community are one of the primary reasons families are referred to his memory care residence. His community has earned a reputation that has many families waiting in line, a situation that many communities would love to have.

Teamwork

In today's workplace, it is rare to see an organization's employees work together as a team. You should expect to see a culture of teamwork in your mom's new community. In my dad's memory care community, the caregivers, medical technicians, maintenance staff, and food staff all seem to have the same mission: How can I help? I've seen the chef sit down with the residents to get to know them. I've seen a medical technician stop to help a resident who needs to be redirected. I've seen other family members stop to spend time with my dad. I've seen caregivers help each and every resident who needs attention. The community you choose should be staffed with employees, top to bottom, that communicate with each other and work together as a team for the common goal—to assist residents.

Activities

The community you choose for your mom should have an activities director that understands the different interests and ability levels of the residents. You might expect to see activities ranging from art, music therapy, bingo, singing, inspirational readings, and special guest visits. The needs of the residents will change as their dementia advances and a skilled activities director will grow familiar with the developing needs within the community. The activity director at my dad's memory care community has been working there for several years and continues to find fresh new ways to engage the residents. In the past year, the activities director has implemented a painting program for the residents that has resulted in colorful art brightening the hallway walls. You should expect the activity director to be accessible. For example, our family wanted to bring in local teenagers to decorate the Christmas tree and to sing holiday songs with the residents. The activity director welcomed the idea and now it's an annual tradition at my dad's community.

Responsiveness

A high-caliber community will be quick to respond to the concerns and suggestions you have for your mom's care. After all, you often know best what Mom needs. My dad had lived his life working as an independent sales person in the financial planning industry. He loved to meet with people and always wanted to help others. When my dad first moved in to his current memory care community he was still walking and active. It was clear that he needed a job to do. I mentioned to Keith that my dad was energetic and loved to work. Right away, Keith and the caregivers began to find ways to give my dad "jobs" to do. On occasion, Keith would let my dad organize nonessential papers on his desk. And, from time to time, one of the caregivers would allow my dad to "go on rounds" to visit residents on the floor. These efforts demonstrated the willingness of the community staff to meet the individual needs of residents and to respond quickly to my dad's needs. That type of responsiveness should be expected in your mom's community.

Medical records access

As the power of attorney for your mom, you have access to her medical records at all times. You should expect her community to allow you to view her records upon request. If you have questions about her medications, changes in behavior, or if there was an event such as a fall that occurred during the night, all of this will be recorded. All medical and care information is required to be documented, and this information belongs to you.

The community and hospice care

If your mom qualifies for hospice (it's not just for end of life), her community should allow hospice care nurses to work with your mom and should view hospice as a secondary layer of care for her. The community should see that the organization holds primary responsibility for Mom and should work with hospice as a team. Keith and his medical director have worked with hospice, but have also consistently taken responsibility to provide care for Mom and Dad, never passing the buck to someone else. And this is the bottom line difference between quality communities and inferior ones: they take ownership of the responsibility to provide quality care. It seems like a logical assumption, but unfortunately many facilities are just kind of a hotel where they provide a room and some basic services, but don't actually provide care and attention.

Final thoughts

If you have an opportunity to find an assisted living or memory care with these qualities—communication that is a top priority at all levels; caregivers dedicated to serving residents and devoted to their job; a community that is in demand; a culture of teamwork; an activities director committed to engaging residents and accessible and open to fresh ideas; a responsiveness and openness to your concerns and requests at every level; open access to medical records; and an attitude of partnership with hospice nurses—then you may have found the right community for Mom.

However, you must always see that Mom's new residence is in fact a place that is partnering with you in her care. You must always be involved in asking questions and paying close attention to the daily and weekly care that Mom is receiving. True care angels are among the most wonderful people you will ever hope to meet. They are filled up and overflowing with compassion, kindness, and a willingness to sacrifice themselves to tackle the difficult task of caring for those who have dementia. However, caregivers are people who aren't always perfect and there will be mistakes from time to time. Visit as much as you can and get to know the caregivers and the other families that are stopping by the community. You may find that your heart is filled up with the happiness and joy that comes from helping others.

13

Financial Solutions

Compared with traditional assisted living or nursing home care, memory care tends to cost more. That's because memory care requires more supervision and caregivers with more advanced skills, especially as dementia progresses. Memory care is typically paid for with private funds. When personal funds can't cover expenses, resources from the government and nonprofit foundations can help meet the need. You may also hire an estate planner, geriatric planner or similar finance expert.

The following are your options for payment/partial payment that most memory care communities accept:

Private Pay - Personal income or savings is the standard route. However, the cost of a month's rent can quickly use up your savings. Often paying out of pocket is beyond what many can afford in the long term. However, when all your resources have been exhausted, you can apply for Medicaid.

Unfortunately, the US government continues to reduce Medicaid programs. Many assisted living communities and memory care communities that at one time accepted Medicaid, no longer can because of the lowered amount that is currently being paid out for senior care. Some states use a Medicaid waiver program in which a set number of residents can be served so there may be a waiting list. At the time of this writing, more "reductions" in Medicaid programs are expected.

Long Term Care Insurance – If Mom has a long-term care policy it will help cover a good portion of the rent and care costs. Most insurance policies are difficult to understand, but knowing your benefits will be helpful in making sure you get what you have paid for. It is common for insurance companies to decline payment on the first go round. On several occasions, I had to contact an insurance company and explain my community's care capabilities and the care plan in order to get approval. To qualify, most insurance companies will require that Mom demonstrates documented assistance with at least two or three Activities of Daily Living (ADL) such as bathing, dressing, transferring, walking and toileting. Long-term care insurance benefits vary widely depending on the policy. Benefits can range from $1,000 to more than $10,000 per month. There are facility-only policies that cover care only in a licensed assisted living facility or skilled nursing facility.

Veterans Benefits (Aid and Attendance) - There is a benefit, known as the Non-Service Connected Improved Pension Benefit with Aide and Attendance that pays toward the cost of assisted living and memory care. This is available to veterans or a surviving spouse who is disabled and whose income is below a certain limit. A veteran must have served at least 90 days on active duty and/or at least one day during wartime. The medical condition doesn't need to be service related, but you must meet medical qualification. There is ever-changing information on exactly how much the government will pay, but the maximum benefit is approximately: $2,120 a month for married veterans, $1,788 for single veterans and $1,149 for a surviving spouse.

Be aware that you may be told that you have too many assets to qualify for this program. What you may not have been told is that you could possibly make some re-allocations or adjustments to your assets without being penalized and then you could qualify. If you need to adjust your assets, I strongly suggest that you contact an Aid and Attendance expert to help you through this process.

Call your local VFW for additional information.

To be eligible for this benefit, one must meet the following requirements:

Age - Veterans or their surviving spouses must be at least 65 or officially disabled if younger.

Period of Military Service - Veterans must be considered wartime veterans meaning they served at least 90 days and served at least 1 day during the wartime dates below, but not necessarily in combat.

> World War II: Dec 7, 1941 – Dec 31, 1946
>
> Korean War: Jun 27, 1950 – Jan 31, 1955
>
> Vietnam War: Aug 5, 1964 – May 7, 1975 (or Feb 28, 1961 – May 7, 1975 for Veterans who served in Vietnam)
>
> Gulf War: Aug 2, 1990 – Undetermined

Discharge Status - Cannot have been dishonorably discharged.

Disability Status - Veterans are eligible without a disability.

Spouse Rules - a surviving spouse must have been married and living with the Veteran at the time of their death. If divorced, the spouse also is divorced from the benefit.

Avoiding Financial Trouble

Shortly after my parents came to live with us, my dad made it clear that he would continue to manage his financial affairs. Moving to a new city was not his idea, and, to him, the entire event felt threatening to his independence. His feelings certainly made sense to everyone in the family as my dad had been earning money since the age of nine when he first took a job during the Depression. That same work ethic carried him through his entire adult career as an independent financial planner. He certainly wasn't ready to let go of the reins any time soon. Out of respect for his wishes, we took steps to protect his finances as well as his pride. Our family agreed that my husband and my brother would sit down with him and discuss his finances to help make sure his affairs were in order. Unfortunately, Dad didn't always remember the discussions he had with them. One day, we discovered that he had paid his income taxes without telling anyone. The big shock came when he paid them twice more. It took several months to get the two overpayments straightened out with the IRS. After more time passed, my dad slowly became adjusted to having his son-in-law and son manage the details of his bills and taxes. It became more important than ever to find other ways for him to use his time. Thankfully, that came in the way of a food outreach program to help feed low-income families. *There's Hope for the Hungry* became a weekly focus that gave my dad a whole new purpose in life.

The key to helping Mom with her finances starts with early conversations. She may be hesitant to let go completely of her financial affairs. Start offering to sit down with her on a regular basis to discuss her finances. You might find that she is relieved to get your input.

–Halle

The following are alternative options for funding Mom's rent and care when private pay is not and option:

<u>Please consult an estate planner or a finance expert before making a decision.</u>

Consider Selling or Renting Your Home – For some families, selling their family home is definitely out of the question. If that's the case, consider renting the home to give you a monthly income that could help with the cost of assisted living or memory care.

Life Insurance Benefits –Life insurance policies that are whole rather than term can be tapped to help pay for memory care. There are three different ways that policies can be used to pay for care while Mom is still alive.

The three options with a whole life policy are: cashing out, selling the policy to a third party, or converting the policy from insurance to long-term care.

Ask your life insurance agent about cashing out the policy, accelerated, or living benefits. It can be called any of those terms. What usually happens is the company will buy the policy back for 50 to 75 percent of its value. Some policies can only be cashed in if the policyholder is terminally ill. If the company won't cash it in, you can sell the policy to a third-party company in return for a life settlement which is usually 50 to 70 percent of the policy face value. After buying the policy, and giving you the percentage, the third-party company continues to pay the premiums until the policyholder dies. At which time, the company receives the benefits. There is also an option called a life insurance conversion program. This allows Mom to switch the benefit of a life insurance policy into long-term care payments. Life insurance conversion typically pays between 15 to 50 percent of the value of the policy. Although this is less than a life settlement, it is an option for lesser-value policies that might not qualify for life settlement.

Bridge Loans - While waiting for the sale of a property or a pension to be approved, a short term loan may help. These loans are usually available up to $50,000 and designed to fund the move to an assisted living or memory care.

Please consult an estate planner or a finance expert before making a decision.

Reverse Mortgage - This allows you to borrow money on the equity you have built up in your home. When the last person is gone from the home, the money needs to be repaid which usually means selling the home. This is definitely not the best choice for a home that you want to keep in the family.

Please consult an estate planner or a finance expert before making a decision.

Grants - National nonprofit organizations give grants for respite care. Some give caregiving funds directly to families. Others grant the funds to local nonprofits and care providers for distribution. To learn more, you can start by contacting the Alzheimer's Foundation of America and the Alzheimer's Association.

Please consult an estate planner or a finance expert before making a decision.

Wisconsin Alzheimer's Family and Caregiver Support Program (AFCSP) - provides respite care services to low and middle income families affected by Alzheimer's disease and other memory disorders. In-home care and adult day care are offered. Unlike with Medicaid, individuals do not need to spend most of their savings to become eligible.

New York Paid Family Leave Benefits Law (PFLBL) - could provide caregiving wages for up to twelve weeks per year, although some employers will opt out.

Alaska Senior In-Home (SIH) Services - program provides daily living assistance to all lowincome state residents ages 60 and older with limited mental or physical capabilities. This program is meant for people who do not qualify for Medicaid but cannot afford to pay privately for care.

California Paid Family Leave (PFL) Act - allows employees to take time off of work (up to six weeks per year) and receive compensation for their caregiving. The wage replacement can equal up to 55 percent of one's job income. This program does not guarantee job security.

Annuity - When Mom has a good deal of money in savings, buying an annuity can help ensure that her savings will last. When you buy an annuity, you pay a lump sum and then receive monthly payments for the rest of your life. The monthly payments might not cover all living expenses, but they ensure regular income nonetheless.

The biggest benefit of an annuity is that even if your purchase premium runs out, you can get more money back than you put in. The underwriters hope to make a profit off you if Mom passes early. They take the risk that Mom could live longer. It can be more beneficial for you than just spending your money on the cost of the stay.

Another advantage of an annuity is that it isn't fully considered an asset by Medicaid when you apply for government assistance. The monthly payment from the annuity is counted as a resource, but the larger sum you originally paid for the annuity is not. This can be tricky, so I strongly recommend you have a reputable accountant, financial adviser or attorney guide you.

Please consult an estate planner or a finance expert before making a decision.

Medicaid - If you have no savings, financial assets, and your income is low, you may qualify for government assistance or Medicaid which is a federal program, but administered by each individual state. Medicaid covers medical benefits for low income citizens with few assets. There is no law, that I am aware of, that requires Medicaid to pay for assisted living. Medicaid approval is based on financial need. They will review your financial transactions for the past five years. If you are caught trying to spend or hide your resources, there are penalties and Mom may be disqualified from receiving Medicaid benefits. Please consult an estate planner or a finance expert before making a decision.

14

What is going on with Mom's memory?

Why is Mom forgetting? One reason is that dementia affects recent memories first and then weakens the retention of new information. New experiences or memories register in the part of the brain called the hippocampus which sends the memory to the brain's memory bank. When Alzheimer's develops, the hippocampus is among the first areas to be damaged. Considering the role of the hippocampus in storing new memories, the affected person is no longer able to recount new information. Alzheimer's affects the brain in such a way that long-term memories will fade over time as well.

The different memory systems include; Episodic, Semantic, Working and Procedural.

Working Memory - Working memory encompasses concentration, keeping attention, and vital information such as a street address or phone numbers. Problems with working memory can weaken Mom's ability to accomplish multi-step tasks.

Procedural Memory - Procedural memory stores information on how to perform many actions, such as walking, jumping, sitting, getting dressed, speaking and even playing piano. It is a part of the long - term memory that is responsible for knowing how to do things, also known as motor skills.

Episodic Memory - The episodic memory is what enables Mom to learn new information and remember new events. The hippocampus is one of the first parts of the brain that is damaged from Alzheimer's. With the passing of time, these changes can make it more difficult for Mom to learn new tasks or to retrieve information from her memory, such as someone's name. Dementia affects recent memories first. The retention of new information is most affected while past memories are much more retrievable.

Semantic Memory - Semantic memory directs wide-ranging knowledge and facts, including the ability to recognize, name, and label objects. Mom may be unable to name a common object or to list objects in a category, such as farm animals or types of birds.

Antoinette

I will always remember a sweet woman who was nearing the final stages of dementia named Antoinette. She would look up at me at least 10 times a day and whisper "I love you." I later learned that she was experiencing a psychological state of euphoria brought on by manic depression. Antoinette spent her days sitting in the front lobby watching people walk by her. If someone would stop and take a moment to smile or say hello, Antoinette would smile back and whisper, "I love you." One day we had a pianist come to perform for the residents. I remember watching the group of ladies in the piano room tapping their feet and bobbing to the music. I noticed Antoinette sitting outside the room fingering keys as she listened to the piano. When the entertainer was finished I walked Antoinette over to the piano and she sat down on the piano stool. I pushed the stool closer to the baby grand and watched her start to play Mozart. The entertainer came back and sat down next to me and just said "Wow!" Residents started walking back into the piano room and sitting down. Antoinette played for about 10 minutes and then stopped. Everyone started applauding, I stood up and walked over to her and told her that her playing was beautiful. She smiled at me and said, "I love you." The next day I called Antoinette's daughter and told her what had happened. Her daughter became very excited and explained that her mother once played at the Metropolitan Opera, but she figured her piano playing days were over.

–Keith

15

Will Mom
Forget Me?

Walking into a room and having your spouse or parent not recognize you can be upsetting and trigger strong emotions.

On occasion, families will unintentionally shower Mom with questions:

"Do you know who I am?"

"Do you remember my wife?"

"Can you tell me my name?"

These types of questions can possibly create more confusion for Mom. A more helpful start to your visit with Mom might be something similar to, "Hi Mom, it's your son Danny." A key to a quality visit is using the following tip: *Explain Everything!*

"Hi Mom, it's your son Danny and I am here to visit you." Be comforting and reassuring, hold Mom's hand, and smile and remind Mom that you are her son. Introduce everyone in your family if needed. Sometimes Mom will say, "Oh, I know all that...thank you for coming."

I love you, babe.

At the age of 89, my dad is now moving toward the later stages of dementia. It's often heart wrenching for me to see him now, a shadow of the strong man I once knew. Memories fill my mind of his younger years when he was the energetic business man, avid sailor, and workout enthusiast. Nearly a year ago he still enjoyed walking the long hallways and courtyard of the community where he lives. Now, he spends long days in his wheelchair and his language is made up of jumbled words that he struggles to deliver. Sometimes he only speaks with his eyes and a squeeze of my hand. Perhaps the words I'll always treasure most are the ones he spoke a few months ago while I sat in the chair beside him and held his hand. He sat quietly and looked at my face with his sparkling blue eyes. We sat together for a long while with no exchange of words. Slowly, he reached up and began to rearrange my hair. I smiled and wondered if, perhaps, he was seeing a younger daughter than the one who sat with him now. I relished the tender moment. Then I said with a big smile, "Dad, I love you." Out of the silence, my precious dad looked at me and said, "I love you, babe."

How thankful I am that I sat and waited in silence, not expecting anything. The waiting rendered a treasure. The best things in life are indeed worth waiting for.

–Halle

To answer the question as to whether or not Mom will forget you, I would say that it is possible that Mom may not have forgotten you and here's why:

Have you ever gone to your high school class reunion? You may have attended your 20- or 30- year reunion. Think about the classmates with whom you reunited. Did you recognize all of them or did you need help recalling some names? There is a reason they make you wear a name tag with your graduation picture on it. Sometimes it takes some time to recognize a former classmate. You look at their eyes, you listen to their voice and you try everything before having to look at their name tag. Does any of this sound familiar?

Think about it: these were important people in your life; you may have spent four years trying to impress these people. Why can't you recognize them now? Did you forget who they are entirely?

Personally, I want to believe that Mom doesn't forget you. I want to think it's possible that Mom just doesn't recognize you. You may have changed quite a bit in the last 20 years and Mom's most vivid memories are 20 to 30 years ago. One day you may come to visit Mom and she doesn't indicate in any way that your presence is known. It may well be that the touch of your hand, your eyes, your hair, the shape of your face, the sound of your voice, or even some sense we cannot understand will connect with her and comfort your mom.

So never give up and always be the best advocate for your loved one.

Notes

Introduction

1. Markham Heid, "Alzhiemer's: A Tutorial," Time Special Edition, The Science of Alzheimer's, May 25, 2018.

2. "Dementia: Key Facts," World Health Organization, http://www.who.int/news-room/fact-sheets/detail/dementia, (accessed January 15, 2018).

Chapter One

1. Jane L. Murphy, Joanne Holmes, and Cindy Brooks, "Nutrition and dementia care: developing an evidence-based model for nutritional care in nursing homes," National Institutes of Health, https://www.ncbi.nlm.nih.gov/pmc/articles/PMC5309970/, (accessed January 15, 2018).

2. "Powers of Attorney: The Basics", National Caregivers Library, http://www.caregiverslibrary.org/caregivers-resources/grp-legal-matters/hsgrp-power-of-attorney-guardianship/powers-of-attorney-theba-sics-article.aspx, (accessed January 16, 2018)

3. "How organ donation works", organdonor.gov, https://www.orgando-nor.gov/about/process.html, (accessed January 13, 2018).

Chapter Two

1. "Dementia Statistics", Alzheimer's Disease International, https://www.alz.co.uk/research/statistics, (accessed January 12, 2018).

2. "Dementia Statistics", Brain Test, https://braintest.com/dementia-stats-u-s worldwide/,(accessed January 12, 2018).

3. "Facts and Figures", Alzheimer's Association, https://www.alz.org/alzheimers-dementia/facts-figures, (accessed January 11, 2018).

4. "Vascular Dementia", Mayo Clinic, https://www.mayoclinic.org/diseases-conditions/vascular-dementia/symptoms-causes/syc-20378793, (accessed January 13, 2018).

5. "Lewy Body Dementia", Mayo Clinic, https://www.mayoclinic.org/diseases-conditions/lewy-bodydementia/symptoms-causes/syc-20352025, (accessed January 10, 2018).

6. "What is Parkinson's?", Parkinson's Foundation, http://www.parkinson.org/understanding-parkinsons/what-is-parkinsons, (accessed January 12, 2018).

7. "Parkinson's Disease: The Incurable Disease," http://tsukinegradprogram.blogspot.com/2016/11/parkinsons-disease-incurable-disease.html, (accessed January 12, 2018).

8. "Frontotemporal dementia." Alzheimer's Society of Canada, http://alzheimer.ca/en/Home/Aboutdementia/Dementias/Frontotemporal-Dementia-and-Pick-s-disease, (accessed January 12, 2018).

9. Michael B. Coulthart, Etal., "A case cluster of variant Creutzfeldt-Jakob disease linked to the Kingdomof Saudi Arabia", https://www.ncbi.nlm.nih.gov/pmc/articles/PMC5082737/. (accessed January 12, 2018).

10. "About Huntington's disease", Alzheimer's Association, https://www.alz.org/alzheimers-dementia/what-is-dementia/types-of-dementia/huntington-s-disease, (accessed January 13, 2018).

11. "Korsakoff syndrome", Alzheimers Association, https://www.alz.org/media/Documents/alzheimersdementia-korsakoff-syndrome-ts.pdf (accessed January 13, 2018).

Chapter Four

12. Sundowning: Late Day Confusion, Mayo Clinic, https://www.mayoclinic.org/diseases-conditions/alzheimers-disease/expert-answers/sundowning/faq-20058511, (accessed January 16, 2018).

Chapter Five

13. "Caregiver Statistics", Family Caregiver Alliance, https://www.caregiver.org/caregiver-statisticsdemographics, (accessed January 16, 2018).

Chapter Ten

14. "Medication Errors: we know they happen", MCN Healthcare, https://www.mcnhealthcare.com/medication-errors/, (accessed January 17, 2018).

Resources

www.assistedlivingtoday.com
www.alz.org
www.premierseniorliving.com
www.caregiverslibrary.org
www.agingcare.com
www.mayoclinic.org
www.healthline.com
www.ncabz.org
www.teepasnow.com
www.secondwind.org
www.curealz.org
www.medindia.net
www.openplacement.com
www.human-memory.net
www.comfortkeepers.com
www.science.howstuffworks.com
www.aplaceformom.com
www.amysplace.net
www.johnscreek-987.comfortkeepers.com
The National Council on Aging Belize
Dementia care at Mayo Clinic
The Alzheimer Society of Canada
The World Alzheimer Report

Studies reviewed for this book:

Prevalence and impact of caregiving: a detailed comparison between dementia and nondementia caregivers.[Gerontologist. 1999] John Hopkins

Family caregiving of persons with dementia: prevalence, health effects, and support strategies. [Am J Geriatr Psychiatry. 2004]

Prevalence and impact of caregiving: a detailed comparison between dementia and nondementia caregivers.[Gerontologist. 1999]

Measuring the wellness of family caregivers using the time trade-off technique.[J Clin Epidemiol. 1988]

Families caring for elders in residence: issues in the measurement of burden [J Gerontol. 1984]

Caregiving and the stress process: an overview of concepts and their measures. [Gerontologist. 1990]

Is the glass half empty or full? Reflections on strain and gain in caregivers of individuals with Alzheimer's disease.[Soc Work Health Care. 2005]

Determinants of burden in those who care for someone with dementia

[Int J Geriatr Psychiatry. 2008]

Coping strategies and anxiety in caregivers of people with Alzheimer's disease: The LASER-AD study [J Affect Disord. 2006]

Determinants of burden in those who care for someone with dementia

[Int J Geriatr Psychiatry. 2008]

Family caregiving of persons with dementia: prevalence, health effects, and support strategies. [Am J Geriatr Psychiatry. 2004]

Stress, appraisal, coping, and social support as predictors of adaptational outcome among dementia caregivers.[Psychol Aging. 1987]

Care arrangements for people with dementia in developing countries.

[Int J Geriatr Psychiatry. 2004]

Emotional adaptation over time in care-givers for chronically ill elderly people [Age Ageing. 1990]

Subjective burden of husbands and wives as caregivers: a longitudinal study [Gerontologist. 1986]

Psychosocial effects on carers of living with persons with dementia [Aust N Z J Psychiatry. 1990]

Predictors of improvement in social support: Five-year effects of a structured intervention for caregivers of spouses with Alzheimer's disease [Soc Sci Med. 2006]

Psychosocial predictors of dementia caregiver desire to institutionalize: caregiver, care recipient, and family relationship factors.[J Geriatr Psychiatry Neurol. 2006]

Psychosocial effects on caregivers of living with persons with dementia

[Aust N Z J Psychiatry. 1990]

Improving caregiver well-being delays nursing home placement of patients with Alzheimer disease.[Neurology. 2006]

Meta-analysis of psychosocial interventions for caregivers of people with dementia.[J Am Geriatr Soc. 2003]

Systematic review of the effect of psychological interventions on family caregivers of people with dementia.[J Affect Disord. 2007]

Systematic review of the effect of psychological interventions on family caregivers of people with dementia.[J Affect Disord. 2007]

A three-country randomized controlled trial of a psychosocial intervention for caregivers combined with pharmacological treatment for patients with Alzheimer disease: effects on caregiver depression.[Am J Geriatr Psychiatry. 2008]

Helping caregivers of persons with dementia: which interventions work and how large are their effects?[Int Psychogeriatr. 2006]

Effect of a training program to reduce stress in carers of patients with dementia.[BMJ. 1989]

Cost effectiveness of a training program for dementia carers.[Int Psychogeriatr. 1991]

Differences between caregivers and non-caregivers in psychological health and physical health: a meta-analysis.[Psychol Aging. 2003]

Enhancing the quality of life of dementia caregivers from different ethnic or racial groups: a randomized, controlled trial.[Ann Intern Med. 2006]

The effectiveness of a home care program for supporting caregivers of persons with dementia in developing countries: a randomized controlled trial from Goa, India [PLoS One. 2008]

Do family caregivers perceive more difficulty when they look after patients with early onset dementia compared to those with late onset dementia? [Int J Geriatr Psychiatry.2007]

Glossary

The following table includes definitions of some of the special language used in senior care.

24-hour Controlled Access	Some senior facilities have security systems that only allow authorized personnel into the buildings.
Activities of Daily Living (ADLs)	Activities of daily living are typically defined as bathing, dressing, assistance with using the toilet, eating, moving around to perform daily life supporting tasks.
Adaptive / Assistive Equipment Definition:	An appliance, gadget or piece of equipment designed to assist users in self-care, leisure activities or work. This can include in-home elevators, special eating implements and walking aids.
Administrator / ED	Typically a licensed professional who has the overall responsibility of the day-to-day operations of a care community like an independent living, assisted living, memory care or nursing home.
Aging in Place	Aging is Place is a concept where seniors continue to live at home or with a family regardless of their mental and physical decline.
Ambulatory	The ability to walk and move freely without assistance, not bedridden or hospitalized.
Activities of Daily Living (ADLs)	Activities of daily living (**ADL**) are routine activities that independent people tend do every day without needing assistance. There are six basic **ADLs**: eating, bathing, dressing, toileting, transferring and continence.
Assessment	An evaluation or test, usually performed by a professional life a physician to determine a person's mental, emotional, and social capabilities.

Case management	A term used to describe a plan of action and care by a professional for a senior or person in need of assistance.
Catheter	A hollow flexible tube for insertion into a body cavity, duct or vessel to allow the passage of fluids or distend a passageway. Catheters are typically used drainage of urine from the bladder through the urethra or insertion through a blood vessel into the heart for diagnostic purposes.
Certificate of Medical Necessity	A document created and signed by an attending physician to certify a patient's need for some type of durable medical equipment (i.e. wheelchairs, walkers, etc.).
RCD (resident care director)	A register nurse (RN) or Licensing Practical Nurse (LPN) who is responsible for the supervision of a Community. The RCD typically schedules and supervises the care staff and provides care to community residents.
Chronic Obstructive Pulmonary Disease (COPD)	A group of chronic respiratory disorders. These disorders are characterized by the restricted flow of air into and out of the lungs like in the case of emphysema.
Cognitive Impairment	A diminished mental capacity. Seniors with cognitive impairment may have difficulty with short-term memory and concentration.
Colostomy	A disposable and replaceable bag is use to for the collection and disposal of bodily wastes.
Congestive Heart Failure (CHF)	A common type of heart disease typically characterized by inadequate pumping action of the heart.
Continuing Care Retirement Community (CCRC)	A community that offers multiple levels of senior living, including independent living, assisted living, hospice and skilled nursing care. A CCRC will create long-term contract between the resident (frequently lasting the term of the resident's lifetime) and the community which offers a continuum of housing, services and health care system throughout the decline of the residence health. All the care options are commonly on one campus or site allow the resident to maintain

Director of Nursing (DON)

Oversees all nursing staff in a nursing home. The DON is responsible for formulating nursing policies and monitoring the quality of care delivered, as well as the facility's compliance with federal and state regulations pertaining to nursing care.

Durable Power of Attorney for Health Care (DPAHC)

A legal document in which a person gives a caregiver (called an attorney-in-fact) the power to make healthcare decisions for him or her if the person is unable to make those decisions. A DPA can include guidelines for the attorney-in-fact to follow in making decisions on behalf of the incompetent person.

E Call System

Some senior care facilities provide a centralized emergency call system such as call buttons in important locations in the unit that allows senior to get emergency help immediately.

Emphysema

One of the two most common forms of chronic obstructive pulmonary disease (COPD). This disorder is based on the obstruction of the bronchial airflow in and out of the lungs. Emphysema is marked by an abnormal accumulation of air in the lung's many tiny air sacs (alveoli). As air continues to collect in these sacs, they become enlarged and may break or be damaged and form scar tissue. The result is labored breathing and an increased susceptibility to infection. Another common COPD is bronchitis.

STR (Short term-Rehabilitation)

Short-term rehabilitation facilities provide therapy for individuals recovering from a surgery, illness or accident. These programs help patients achieve their maximum functional capacity and safely return home in the shortest time possible. To achieve this goal, patients receive physical, occupational and speech therapy from compassionate and highly skilled therapists.

HHC (Home Health Care)

Home health care helps older adults live independently for as long as possible, even with an illness or injury. It covers a wide range of services and can often delay the need for more supportive forms of housing, such as assisted living. Services frequently include occupational, physical and speech therapies as well as nursing care.

Elopement	When a resident leaves the communities property unsupervised. Exit seeking refers to a resident that is looking for a way to get outside.
Respite Care	Respite care is designed to provide temporary relief for those who have the responsibility of caring for a senior family member. It is known that providing such care may result in increasing the caregiver's fatigue and anxiety, impairing the caregiver's ability to function effectively.
NOC	Meaning nocturnal, the term NOC is used in a variety of ways. A NOC nurse would be the nurse who is on shift at night. You will see this term most often in charting and physician orders. This term is also used to describe a level of care if a patient is needing care at night
q. h.	As seen on a prescription bottle, q.h. is derived from the Latin quaque (every) and hora (hour). E.g., if the prescription reads, "2 caps q3h" that means the patient is to take 2 capsules every 3 hours.

Community Tour Score

Let's give it a score so we can compare with other locations.
Rate each category with a score 0 - 5

Community Name _____   Community Name _____

Apartment _____   Apartment _____

Staff_____   Staff_____

Amenities_____   Amenities_____

Location_____   Location_____

Medical_____   Medical_____

Rent/Fees___ x 1.5 ( ) __   Rent/Fees___ x 1.5 ( ) __

Score Total _____   Score Total _____

Community Name _____   ## Example

Apartment _____   Apartment ____5__ Perfect

Staff_____   Staff_____4__ Very Nice

Amenities_____   Amenities_____4__ Great

Location_____   Location_____5__ 2 Miles Away

Medical_____   Medical_____5__ Great Survey

Rent/Fees___ x 1.5 ( ) __   Rent/Fees__5 x 1.5 (7.5) Under Budget

Score Total _____   Score Total ___30.5__

Notes_____

_____

_____

_____

PDF available at www.parentaldementia.com

VALUE GRAGH

How important is it to you?

Questions	Not				Very
To live as long as possible, regardless of quality of life	1	2	3	4	5
To be as comfortable and as pain-free as possible	1	2	3	4	5
To **not** be kept alive by life support	1	2	3	4	5
To leave good memories for family and friends	1	2	3	4	5
To make a contribution to medical research	1	2	3	4	5
To be able to leave money to family, friends, charity	1	2	3	4	5
To **not** have a feeding tube?	1	2	3	4	5
To **not** be given CPR?	1	2	3	4	5
To **not** be given Chemotherapy?	1	2	3	4	5
To be an organ donor?	1	2	3	4	5
Where you have your funeral	1	2	3	4	5
Where you are buried	1	2	3	4	5
Where your ashes are kept	1	2	3	4	5
To have Family by your side when the time comes	1	2	3	4	5
To have religious advisors by your side when the time comes	1	2	3	4	5
That your loved ones know your wishes, values and beliefs?	1	2	3	4	5

Notes

PDF available at www.parentaldementia.com

https://www.aarp.org/caregiving/financial-legal/free-printable-advance-directives

Types Of Dementia	Onset	Explanation	Symptoms
Alzheimer's	Progressive	Develops as a vicious cycle of Abeta peptide accumulation, nerve cell death and inflammation. Eventual nerve cell death	Agitation, Depression, Anxiety, Abnormal motor behavior, Elated mood, Irritability, Apathy, Impulsivity, Delusions (often believing people are stealing from them) and hallucinations Changes in sleep and/or appetite.
Vascular	Gradual	Multi-infarct dementia; dementia due to single infarcts; dementia due to diffuse white matter damage.	Cognitive, motor, and behavioral.
Lewy Body	Progressive quick progression.	Malfunctions in the Autonomic Nervous System.	Parkinson's symptoms, such as a hunched posture, balance problems and rigid muscles. Visual hallucinations. REM sleep disorders.
Frontotemporal "Pick's disease"	Progressive quick progression.	Frontal lobe and/or anterior temporal lobe atrophy.	Loss of Memory, perception, personality changes and speech difficulties. Deep deficiencies in executive functioning and working memory.

WORKSHEET

Family Duties

Proxy_____

Visits_____
_____
_____
_____

Medications
_____
_____
_____
_____
_____
_____

Emergency Calls
1st _____

2nd _____
_____

Transportation
_____
_____
_____

Doctors
_____
_____
_____

Hair_____
Food_____
_____

ICD_____
_____

Pet Care
_____
_____
_____

Advance Directives

_____   Living Will

_____   POA

_____   DNR

_____   POLST/MOLST

_____   Donation

_____   Values

Caregivers
_____
_____
_____
_____

Home Care Companies
_____
_____
_____

Community Tours
_____
_____
_____
_____
_____

Referral Services
_____
_____
_____

Attorneys
_____
_____
_____

Insurance
_____
_____

Hospital of Choice
_____
_____

Monthly Budget

Homecare
_____

Daycare
_____

Daycare with Homecare
_____
_____

Assisted Living
_____

Memory Care
_____
_____

PDF available at www.parentaldementia.com

Despite our most careful planning, the
Road of Life is unpredictable.

*Life is what happens
while you are busy
making other plans*

–John Lennon

"Mann Tracht, Un Gott Lacht"